ADDICTIONS AND BUPRENORPHINE

ADDICTIONS AND BUPRENORPHINE

Cesar A. Fabiani, MD., DLFAPA

To order additional copies of this book, contact:
Xlibris Corporation
1-888-795-4274
www.Xlibris.com
Orders@Xlibris.com
110423

Contents

The Celtic Cross

The Celtic cross (1) at the cover of this book is the symbol of eternity and freedom. This ringed cross is much a symbol of ethnic heritage as it is of faith. It emphasizes the endlessness of God's love as shown through Christ's sacrifice on the cross, topped by a white peace dove. It was given to me by one of my patients. I keep it to remind me of faith, freedom, eternity, and peace when I am dealing with persons who are suffering this serious chronic brain disorder we call addiction.

To my patients. To whom I own my inspiration. Without it, this book could not have been written.

Faith as a moving force

Nothing in life is more wonderful than faith—the one great moving force which we can neither weigh in the balance nor test in the crucible.

—*The Life of Sir William Osler*, Vol. II, 222

INTRODUCTION AND DEFINITIONS

Let's forgive and carry on, continue together for the peace of Colombia.

—Sebastian Escobar

In the film *Sins of My Father*, the son of Pablo Escobar, Sebastian Escobar, tells the infamous and incredible story of his father, the boss of Colombia's Medellin drug cartel, and asks forgiveness from the sons of one of Pablo Escobar's many victims. Similarly we should ask for forgiveness while endorsing the criminality of individuals with drug addiction and treating them with a medical model. This is the goal of this book. Further, in the above mentioned movie, Sebastian states that the drug dealing money was useless. Running out of food, he and his family were surrounded by millions of dollars that they had to use as fuel to warm themselves up. They couldn't use the money to buy rice across the street because the police was there next door to the grocery store, waiting for them to catch them up! He and the Pablo Escobar victims made a very emotional scene and made peace, which allow him to live in Argentina and have a community productive life for himself and his family.

I wish we have the same peace with drug addicted persons, treating them not as criminals but as persons who are victims of a disease and applying a humane medical model to treat them. From a political point of view, drug dealing continues to cause despair and suffering to millions of individuals.

Let us just remind ourselves of the war with drug dealers that is right now taking place in Mexico.

However, from a scientific point of view, the panorama is very different and optimistic if we understand addictions with a medical model, as a disease of the brain that can be prevented and treated.

This book is a summary of my experience of forty years as an addiction psychiatry specialist as well as some thoughts about "astral traveling" or "spirituality" (astral = "related to sacred matters, incorporeal, rather than lay or temporal") (2), which is related to psychological treatments of addictions with the mobilization of unknown neurotransmitters. These thoughts are based on my father's life endeavor with the occult and Masonry, which inspire me to become a doctor in medicine. Furthermore, I think the mobilization of paranormal or occult forces may have some practical value such as acupuncture as part of the biopsychosocial model in the treatment and prevention of addictions.

Addictions

The term *addictions* (I use the plural noun because persons always have more than one addiction) will replace dependence in the DSM-5. This term's etymological origin is from the Latin *addicere*. In Rome, it was given to conquered slaves. They were addicted to the Roman Empire (3). It encapsulates the essence of addictions: lack of freedom to make choices. The treatment of addictions is to make a person free to make choices, with the faith symbolized in the Celtic cross, and spirituality that many recovering persons experience ideally helps a person to maintain sobriety. Although, and due to comorbidities (more than one disease and not just addictions), this goal is complicated but not impossible to achieve.

In the recent epidemic to opiate addictions, evidence based medicine suggests that maintenance therapy is the most successful type of therapy for opiate addictions. Maintenance of either methadone or, in my opinion, when you have chosen the right patient, buprenorphine. The underlying concept is that addicted persons genetically lack certain neurotransmitters. They self-medicate usually with the wrong chemical. Buprenorphine, which is a partial opiate agonist, is the closest to the ideal medication. Partial opiate agonist means that it has a ceiling dose of 32 mg (at 16 mg, 86 percent of all the opiate brain receptors are occupied with buprenorphine). Above this dose, it is not effective (in my opinion, except for the treatment of comorbid pain in which higher than 16 mg dosages may be needed). In other words, it cannot produce respiratory depression. Consequently, nobody can die from an overdose. That is, if it is not mixed with other addictive substances. Nevertheless it is not a magic pill, but close to it! As many addicted persons state, "Now I can function normally." Another very important part of the biopsychosocial model in the treatment of opiate addiction is psychotherapy, counseling, and attending self-help meetings. Here is where spirituality and astral forces come to play a crucial part of its treatment.

Figure 1

ADDICTIONS
THE BIOPSYCHOSOCIAL MODEL

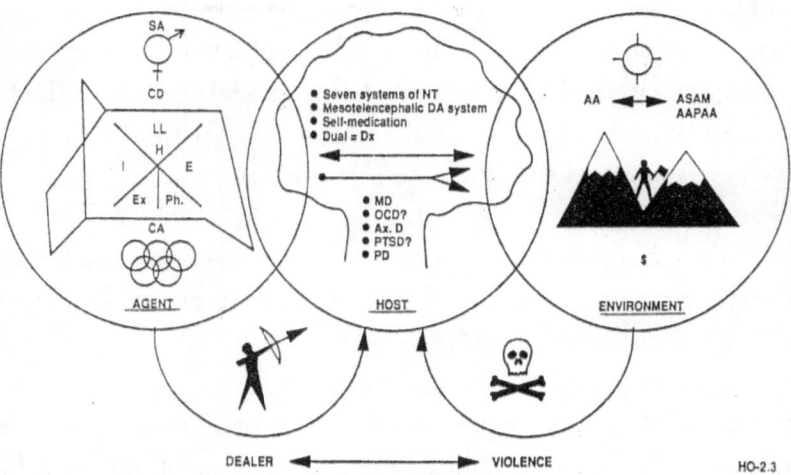

A more scientific definition of addiction is a biopsychosocial one (Figure 1). It overlaps the public health model of agent (biological), host (psychological), and environment (social).

"The self-induction (psychological aspect) in an attempt to correct the genetical lack of certain neurotransmitters" in the "pleasure centers of the brain" (biological aspect), which causes bad social consequences (social aspect), (4) these tree aspects are equally important.

The origin of this important model is the systems theory and the works of Weiss (5) and von Bertalanffy (6). This theory establishes the existence of systems with hierarchy. It starts with atoms, ascending to molecules, cells, tissues, organs, systems, persons or individuals, family, society, and universe. The person is the one who has progressed the most among biological entities and the lowest in the social system. Each system is connected and has a reciprocal interaction with the others. Von Bertalanffy defined this theory as "a system with parts in reciprocal interaction." It was the internist, Dr. George Engel, (7) in 1977, who as professor of medicine and psychiatry in the University of Rochester in New York, presented this biopsychosocial model to replace the biomedical model in medicine and has become so popular specially in psychiatry, perhaps because psychiatry has always emphasized the importance of psychosocial factors in the pathogenesis of illness. He illustrated the clinical application of this model with a patient who in six months has two myocardial infarcts; this patient's therapeutic management improved with the active participation of his wife.

The DSM-IV definition of drug dependence (8) states that if you have three out of seven symptoms, you have dependence. In summary, I encapsulate these symptoms with the three C's.

Control (loss of it). Once you start to take the drug or other agents such as food in eating disorders, gambling in pathological gambling, or Internet, you lose the control and do more and more to the dangerous point of OD (overdose) or other destructive consequences.

Compulsion. You have to do it over and over, many more times.

Consequences. Despite negative biopsychosocial consequences, you cannot stop. If you have had a lung removed due to cancer due to smoking, you continue smoking tobacco. If you get depressed, suicidal, or paranoid due to using cocaine, you continue doing it. If you have wasted thousands of dollars buying opiates, if you have had several DUI due to driving under the influence of alcohol or other dangerous drugs or other serious legal problems, you do not stop but continue doing it.

A more comprehensive definition of addictions as a primary chronic brain disease (9) was published after consulting with more than eighty experts in the field on April 12, 2011, by ASAM (American Society of Addiction Medicine), more than twenty years after the AMA (American Medical Association) in 1990 defined alcoholism as a disease. These definitions are very important because they combat the stigma against addiction. One important fact about this definition is that it encompasses more than the neurochemistry of reward. A fact that we knew long time ago: the brain works in orchestration of many neurochemical systems. The frontal cortex of the brain and underlying white matter connections and circuits of reward, motivation, and memory are fundamental in the manifestations of altered neurochemistry, impulse control, altered judgment, and the dysfunctional pursuit of reward seen in addictions. In this definition, addiction is characterized by five important symptoms:

1. Inability to consistently abstain
2. Impairment in behavioral control
3. Craving or increased "hunger" for drug or rewarding experiences
4. Diminished recognition of significant problems with one's behaviors and interpersonal relationships (importance of spiritual experiences?) and
5. A dysfunctional emotional response.

This definition ends with "recovery from addiction is best achieved through a combination of self-management, mutual support (spiritual factors), and professional care provided by trained and certified professionals." I think this is too long of a definition but a comprehensive one. Again let me repeat that these definitions have a very important goal: an antidote against the stigma of addictions.

Astral

According to the *Webster* dictionary(10), "Theosophy: consisting of, belonging to or being a supersensible substance supposed to be next above the tangible world in refinement." It comes from the Latin *astralis* meaning "of or relating to the stars, or thought coming from the stars." Astral travel is often known as an out-of-body experience. According to some occult explanations, there is an astral nonphysical body next to the physical one. The conscious separation of both would be astral travel. In this book, I will use *astral* as synonymous to *spiritual*, just as an attempt to put together what we know and we do not know that well.

However, as I stated before, my interest in astral travel comes from my father's unpublished manuscript "Spiritual Chats" (11). Despite my father's occupation as an architect, he devoted all his life and forty years of experience to know more about the occult and Masonry (he was the great master and founder of the lodge Nosce Te Ipsum (Inner Self-Knowledge) on September 18, 1953, in Cochabamba, Bolivia; its fiftieth anniversary was celebrated in the year 2003). This obsession of his motivated and inspired me to study medicine and then psychiatry. It was in Cordoba, Argentina, while as a medical student, rotating in the Institute of Alcoholism, that I "cured" an alcoholic patient just with my advice: telling him that in order to save his life and his family, he must stop drinking. He remained sober. It worked! He quit drinking. Obviously something else, healthy spiritual and neurochemical changes in the patient's brain (?) beside my advice, took place. This patient's grateful family gave me chickens as a present. This simple fact motivated my interest in the field of addictions.

Figure 2

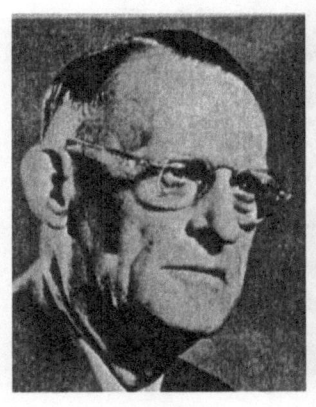 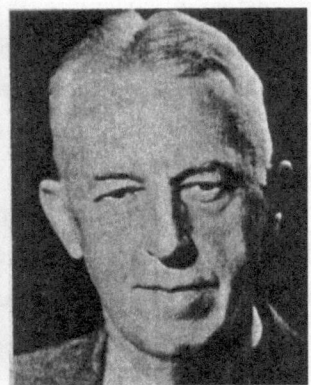

Dr. Bob   Bill W.

Another connection between spirituality, astral knowledge, and addictions comes from the "spiritual awakening" experienced by the founders of AA (12), Bill Wilson, a stockbroker, and Dr. Bob Smith (Figure 2), a surgeon, who on June 10, 1935, quit drinking and founded AA in Akron, Ohio. Both founded this important and universal organization. As a classmate of Dr. Smith, Professor Watson puts it, "A great reformer of himself and others, we feel proud to have had as our classmate, Dr. Robert Hoolbrook Smith. His influence has been spread all over our planet." Dr. Smith and Wilson's "spiritual awakening" must have some neurochemical explanation as well as a spiritual and astral one, which we do not know enough about yet.

However, we should give credit where credit is due. According Bill Wilson, the origins of AA are traced back to Carl Jung, famous Swiss psychoanalyst. Jung had stated to an American alcohol-addicted person, Rowland H. a well-to-do person from Vermont that his knowledge of psychoanalysis was useless against alcoholism, but he offered hope "if he (Rowland H.) experienced a spiritual transformation." Rowland decided to look for this spiritual "awakening" and found it in a spiritual and popular movement in Europe and the USA in 1932: the so-called Oxford Group. Attending one of its meetings in New York, Rowland met a countryman from Vermont, Edwin T. ("Ebby"). Both helped each other with this simple formula of "helping each other." No doubt as part of their "<u>spiritual awakening</u>," they had some astral experiences. What neurotransmittrers but dopamine, serotonin, and endorphines were surely mobilized into a balanced state? They learned to correct their mistakes using meditation and changing into altruistic and generous persons. The connection with Dr. Bob Smith goes back to December 11, 1934, when Wilson was hospitalized for alcohol detox at Towns Hospital in Brooklyn, New York; there he was visited by Ebby. After this visit, Wilson experienced a <u>spiritual awakening</u> that miraculously stopped his obsession for alcohol. Once released from the hospital, he was given advice by Dr. William Silkworth, "the doctor who gave hope to alcoholics," to continue his spiritual experiences, which he did by speaking to other alcoholics; instilling faith and hope to others, he helped himself. One of the "others" was the surgeon, Dr. Bob Smith, who was at the verge of losing his medical license. Their inspiring and immortal experience took place in Akron, Ohio, where Bill was down the dumps due to a setback in business, in an attempt to drown his sorrows in alcohol. He looked up the phone book, looking for a member of the Oxford group; he talked to Henrietta Seiberling who was not an alcoholic. She realized immediately Bill's needs and arranged the historic meeting with Dr. Bob Smith, a brilliant surgeon but going down professionally. Dr. Bob Smith, with second thoughts, reluctantly accepted to talk to Bill. Ironically Dr. Smith was also from Vermont. Both helped themselves despite their shakes from alcohol withdrawal; their meeting lasted nine hours and was the beginning of AA. Dr. Smith relapsed a few days later in a medical convention in Atlantic City, however, due to another "<u>spiritual awakening</u>" experience, quit for good on June 10,1935, the day on which the worldwide anniversary of AA foundation is celebrated.(13) The secret of their success has to be the mobilization of neurotransmitters and astral and spiritual forces among the members who get sober and maintain their sobriety for the rest of their lives helping others. No more altruistic and generous goal could exist.

In 1939, their first one hundred members decided to publish a book that has been disseminated all over the world, *Alcoholic Anonymous.* In July 1985,

AA celebrated their golden anniversary. In 1983, in Los Angeles, an AA member (14) who worked in the movie industry was touched by the cocaine epidemic. He consequently founded CA (Cocaine Anonymous) in an effort to help so many persons addicted to cocaine. Together with NA (Narcotic Anonymous), they cover the pharmacology of the most important addictive drugs. Their message the sine qua non for the polysubstance addiction is "total abstinence" from all addictive substances. Inspired by these historically very important events in Huntington Hospital, Pennsylvania, I founded the first group of Cocaine Anonymous in Pennsylvania on March 5, 1986.

Acupuncture

Acupuncture is a therapy developed by the ancient Chinese that consists of stimulating designated points on the skin by the insertion of needles, which allows a healthy and balanced distribution of electric energy. It also involves application of heat (moxibustion), massage (finger pressure or shiatsu massage), or a combination of these. Acupuncture is part of the overall system of Chinese medicine. For this reason, the Western literature on acupuncture and addiction is scarce. However, Dr. Robert Clark, a good friend and colleague of mine, while being the medical director of Harlem Hospital in New York, used it very successfully among addicted patients. He says, "They (addicted patients) will come from farther away just to get their session of acupuncture." His program was terminated when the grant that sponsored it terminated. Something similar happened in Philadelphia at Girard Medical Center. Since acupuncture is not reimbursed by CBH (Community Behavioral Health), it is not being used. Nonetheless, with the help of Dr. Clark as our consultant at APM (Association of Puerto Ricans in March) and the help of the Philadelphia Office of Addictions Services headed by Roland Lamb, MA, *also Adolfo Gonzalez* and Cheryl Pope, PhD, deputy vice president of human services at APM, we are writing a grant proposal to use acupuncture among Latino patients at APM. No doubt in my mind that acupuncture has to stimulate spiritual, astral centers and chakras with increased neurotransmitters such us adrenaline, testosterone, serotonin, dopamine and endorphins, and others. This therapy will benefit not only patients who are addicted and going through withdrawal but the depression and anxiety of many Latino patients among whom these disorders are pandemic such as the case of PTSD (postraumatic stress disorder) and other anxiety disorders such as panic disorder, MDD (major depressive disorder), bipolar disorders, and addictions.

Comorbidity

> The whole should be known and treated. If we do not treat the
> whole, the parts will not get better.
>
> —Plato

Comorbidity or "dual diagnosis, co-occurring disorders" (Figure 3) are associated diagnosis to addictions; it must be specified if they are medical or psychiatric.

Figure 3

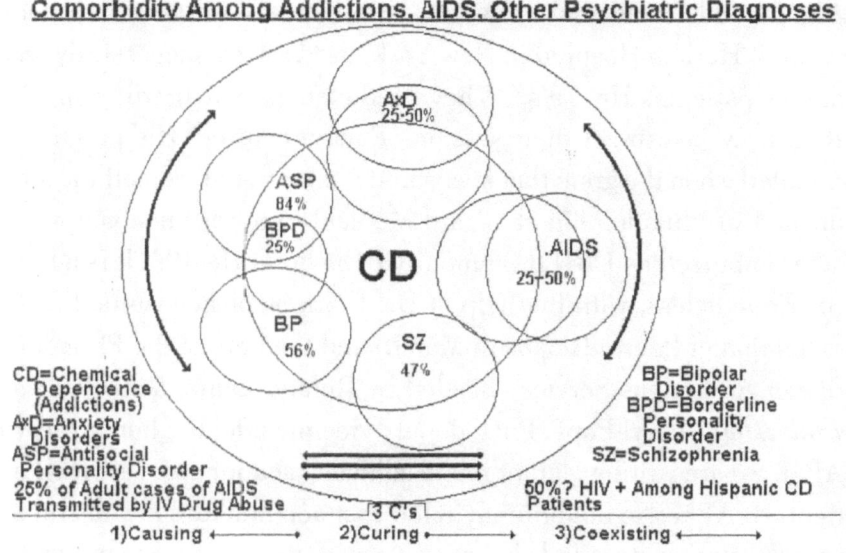

Comorbidity Among Addictions, AIDS, Other Psychiatric Diagnoses

An example would be a Latino patient who has the following diagnoses: addiction to opiates, nicotine, alcohol, and Internet; also borderline personality disorder, bipolar disorder NOS, PTSD, migraine headaches, type II diabetes, obesity, hypertension—eleven diagnoses!

I use *comorbidity* when in addition to addictions, the patient has other diagnoses on Axis I, II, III of the DSM-IV. This is more the rule than the exception. The original term was "dual diagnoses" applied to psychiatric patients who had mental retardation and other psychiatric diagnoses, such as schizophrenia and mental retardation (propfschizophrenia); then it was applied to addictions and other psychiatric diagnoses, but it implied a false dichotomy, between addictions and other psychiatric diagnoses,if medical diagnoses were added for instance addictions and AIDS or head injuries; dual diagnoses became "triple or quadruple diagnoses," obviously a confusing terminology. However, I realized then in the decades of the eighties and nineties this was very common. An integrated treatment program was necessary. As such, we began to establish treatment programs where all these diagnoses could be addressed. First in APM, we made the first simple epidemiological study among Latino patients. It was found that about 50 percent of patients who attended the mental health clinics had addictions (15). Later in Girard Medical Center, we created the first Latino inpatient project for this type of patients (16).

HISTORY OF ADDICTIONS IN GENERAL

Certain people use certain substances in certain ways thought at certain times to be unacceptable by certain people for reasons both certain and uncertain.

—Burglass and Shaffer

Addictions are as old as mankind. Most of them are related to drugs. Nonetheless a nonchemical type of getting high is the Internet and to spin around, which children discover early in childhood. This high is found in a more graphic and impressive form in the dervish dancing in Egypt and other Middle Eastern countries. A dervish is a member of any of various Muslim ascetic orders, some of whom perform whirling dances in ecstatic devotion.

However, chemical addiction refers to the excessive consumption of natural substances such as alcohol, cocaine, cannabis, hallucinogens, hot peppers (now so popular worldwide but indigenous to Bolivia (17)), tobacco, and opium. All of the above will produce a "natural high" not always harmful if used in moderation by the release in the CNS of endorphins.

Notwithstanding, nicotine is the most common legal addiction in the USA. Currently there are at least 50 million people addicted to smoking or chewing tobacco. The most common illegal drug is marijuana. A recent Gallup poll revealed that for the first time in their history, 50 percent of Americans believe marijuana should be legalized. "It is what you might call an all-time high." (18) Along these lines, Burgless's definition of *addictions* is quite apropos. Sixteen states have legalized medicinal use "medical marijuana" like California and New Jersey. Of course, the laws and regulations governing medical marijuana vary from state to state. In California, it is creating a lot of controversy because of its abuse. (19) Adults who obtain a recommendation from a physician is based on the determination "that the person's health would benefit from the use of marijuana in the treatment of cancer, anorexia, AIDS, chronic pain, spasticity, glaucoma, arthritis, migraine, or any other illness for which marijuana provides relief." However, no state has legalized marijuana for recreational purposes. Let's recall that the most common psychoactive substance is caffeine. Caffeine has been proven to have antidepressant effects in women (20). Caffeine released neurotransmitters such as dopamine and serotonin; this is the explanation of its antidepressant effects. However, persons have also reported it can trigger off panic attacks if drinking more than five cups (250 mg/kg) of strong coffee. Moderation is the name of the game.

Let's make it clear that the legal use of these illegal drugs is reserved for persons who do not have addiction. That is why this diagnosis is important.

Although I am going to stress the neurochemical aspects of addiction, the social aspects are as important.

Burglass and Shaffer, in the 1981 definition of addictions stated above, tells me that all depends on your sample and the environment where they take place. Cigarette was considered a "movie-glamour drug" in the thirties, forties, and fifties until we now know some of its harmful effects. Nothing to say about the financial aspects of it. In a recent TV show, *Injustice* (21), some of this money aspects are illustrated by the not very honest lawyers, "tort kings," such as Dick Scruggs who was sent to jail in 2008 after proving that he had made about 200 billion dollars with lawsuit settlements since 1964. First the tobacco lawyers of Mississippi, which spread throughout the rest of the country, then asbestosis and silicosis up to Wall Street law, all of them suit settlements, and many of them perhaps superfluous if not fraudulent.

They considered a lawsuit similar to a three-legged stool: one, the law, the other leg, politics, and the final leg, public relations. That is why only 15 percent of Americans in general trust lawyers.

Cannabis is almost legal in many Muslim countries. Opium/cocaine the same. Opposite sides of the same coin. It all depends on what you are specifically talking about, but we cannot generalize. No doubt that cocaine snorting or smoking are addictive but how about coca-leaves chewing? We just do not know enough. The Surgeon General Dr. C. Everett Koop started his public health efforts in 1984, establishing that smoking can cause lung cancer, and the prevalence of smoking went down among men from 51.9 percent to 28.1 percent in 1991. Diabetes and obesity are among the most devastating illnesses that override tobacco. However, we estimate than in the year 2011 only about 10 percent of men are addicted to tobacco, not a small achievement. There are seven medications approved for the treatment of nicotine addiction. However, the crucial question is, which treatment works better for whom? Nonetheless now opioids. What other drugs will be more prevalent after the year 2012? As long as we do not apply the medical model to treat addictions, the pendulum will be oscillating back and forth.

The IOM (Institute of Medicine) is actively working in establishing health parameters for the year 2011. Health measures and health outcomes in youth. Health-based measures of fitness are those that are most meaningful for monitoring and improving health.

For the past three decades, the Department of Health and Human Services (DHHS) has issued a national agenda aimed at improving the health of all Americans over each ten-year span. With this basis, the IOM identified a set of basic principles for Healthy People 2020 and developed a conceptual framework, motivating diverse population groups to engage in activities that will exert a positive impact on specific indicators and, in turn, improve the overall health of the nation.

I will review some history pertinent to alcohol, cocaine, and opiates as well as neurochemistry, clinical aspects and treatment. I will first illustrate some positive effects of these drugs that apply only to the nonaddicted person.

ALCOHOL ADDICTION

The abuse of wine cause many symptoms of insanity. These
abuses cause half of cases seen in England. In Pennsylvania
according Dr. Rush, it is also a common cause of insanity.
—E. Esquirol, *Mental Maladies* (1845)

History

From a practical point of view, with the exception of the Muslim countries,
alcohol is the most common psychotropic drug, second only to caffeine,
and the oldest drug in our planet. I will state some positive effects of
both caffeine and alcohol. Regarding alcohol, its positive effects among
persons who are not addicted to it is that it is a good vasodilator. Only in
an emergency and for a short time and when no other medications such
as benzodiacepines are available, it could prevent delirium tremens. It is
also proven that in moderation, it has a "social lubricant effect," promoting
social interaction. Alcohol also increases the levels of good cholesterol. By
moderation, I refer to not more than 1-2 drinks (an ounce of liquor proof,
a normal glass of wine or beer) daily among women and men respectively.
Regarding caffeine, it is the most popular stimulant available worldwide.
It may also have some antidepressant effects as stated above.

Written records of alcohol use are found in Chinese and Middle Eastern
texts as far back as nine thousand years ago. The *Triumph of Bacchus*

(22), Diego Rodriguez De Silva y Velazquez's (1599-1660) painting of Bacchus, is the most popular mythological work that illustrates the mixed blessing and curse that alcohol brings to humanity. Bacchus offered the first grape plants for cultivation to help a poor but noble farmer whom he befriended. All went pretty well for the farmer until some of his neighbors got drunk and, thinking they have been poisoned, killed him. Bacchus too was sometimes driven out of his mind by its excessive use. Moderation is the name of the game.

Recent studies suggest that "alcohol is more dangerous than illegal drugs like heroin and crack cocaine." This study comes from the Lancet. "Alcohol scored so high because it is so widely used and has devastating consequences not only for the drinker but for those around him." (23)

In 2006, excessive drinking cost $223.5 billion. This study appeared in the American Journal of Preventive Medicine. That amounts to $750 for every person in the country or about 1.90 per drink. Almost one-third of the $223.5 billion were tied to loses in workplace activity (72 percent) followed by health-care expenses (11 percent), law enforcement and criminal justice expenses (9 percent) and other effects. In this study, Ms. Bauchery and her colleges defined binge drinking (four or more drinks for a woman and five or more per man) and heavy drinking (more than one drink per day on average per woman and more than two per man). They found that about $94.23 billion (42 percent) of the total costs were borne by federal, state, and local government. While $92.9 billion was borne by excessive drinkers and their families, most of the costs due to loss of productivity (55 percent) primarily in the way of lower household income. Most of binge drinkers are not alcoholic. There are many scientifically proven strategies that can reduce excessive drinking; doctors, nurses, and other health-care professionals can intervene to advice patients in ways that will reduce their progress to harmful drinking over time. This is a good and simple way of prevention.

From the medical point of view, in the USA, the first one to consider alcoholism as a medical disorder was the father of American psychiatry, Benjamin Rush (24) who in 1785 wrote a book, *An Inquiry into the Effects of Ardent Spirits upon the Human Body and Mind.* In a thermometer, he described the harmful effects of alcohol in the body. It was a list of medical complications as well as punishments. It was the English physician E. Trotter (25) who in 1804 established alcoholism as a disease. However, the classic book was written in 1960 by the Swedish alcoholism pioneer E. M. Jellinek, *The Disease Concept of Alcoholism* (26). He described four types of alcoholism designated with the Greek alphabet. He was ahead of his times and thought that a genetic factor X predisposed to the development of these different types of alcoholism. A landmark in this field was Magnus Huss's 1849 publication of his text "Chronic Alcoholism." It contributed with the acceptance of the term *alcoholism.* Quoting Huss, "These symptoms are formed in such a particular way that they form a disease group in themselves and thus merit being designated and described as a definite disease . . . It is these group of symptoms which I wish to designate by the name Alcoholismus chronicus." (27)

The AMA in 1968 acknowledged alcoholism as a disease, (28) describing it as chronic, progressive, incurable (a patient cannot go back to "normal" drinking. A normal life may resume but only with the permanent and complete abstinence from alcoholic beverages), with loss of control over drinking.

There are "normal" drinkers, about 43 percent of US adults. Seventy-six million people have been exposed to alcohol. In these normal drinkers, alcohol may even have some salutary effects, for instance, increasing the "good" cholesterol HDL. Nevertheless, I will refer to nearly 14 million Americans who have problems with drinking. More than half of them (9.8 million) may be alcoholic. The prevalence of alcoholism has to be taken with a grain of salt. All depends on your sample.

Among Latinos, their prevalence is one of the highest, 34 percent in Mexican Americans. On the other hand, alcoholism prevalence among women in Peruvians and Puerto Ricans is one of the lowest at 2.46 percent.(29)

In Bolivia, alcoholism is a pandemic, in my estimate and depending on the sample, almost 30 percent due not only to genetics but also to cultural factors as Kuczynski-Godard stated (30), "Indian life has three important cultural escapes: migration to escape from your poverty, coca-leaves to camouflage hunger, and alcohol to forget your social misery." This social misery with the first Indian president in Bolivia has changed into ignorant rebellion trying to expand the plantation of coca-leaves. This statement has to be taken with a grain of salt.

The distinction between considering alcoholism as a disease and not a moral flaw is very important one. It is very useful to combat the tremendous stigma in the past associated with alcoholism. The more aware the public is that alcoholism is a disease like hypertension or diabetes, the less stigma. The more prevention and treatment is possible. As a colleague stated, "It is the most treatable but untreated disease." It contributes to one hundred thousand deaths annually, making it the third leading cause of preventable mortality. For instance, studies of suicide victims in the general population show that about 20 percent are alcoholic. However, 80 percent of people who faithfully attend AA meeting for two years are abstinent after ten years! Success more than in the treatment of hypertension or diabetes!

Bolivian alcoholic tetany illustrates the role of the environment in alcoholism. In Bolivia, I described an alcoholic syndrome that has not been previously reported in medical literature (31-32-33). It resembles tetany. The vernacular and colloquial name is *tistapis*, which in the Aymara language means "cramps."

It seems to be indigenous to Bolivia. Tistapis or Bolivian alcoholic tetany is seen only above thirteen thousand feet above sea level. Around La Paz,

Bolivia, it has an incidence of 10-15 percent mostly among alcohol-addicted persons. This syndrome presents itself as part of the alcohol withdrawal syndrome.

A brief description of a patient with tistapis follows. A forty-four-year-old male of mixed Indian and Spanish bred, born in Potosi. He was admitted with the diagnosis of alcohol dependence and "alcoholic neuropathy" (which is the wrong and most common diagnosis of this syndrome). Onset of tistapis came after an alcohol binge of seven consecutive days of drinking sugarcane alcohol diluted with water. The patient, after six hours of stopping drinking alcohol. He experienced intense and very painful cramps, thirst, hand tremors, insomnia, and severe depressive mood mixed with anxiety. The cramps involved upper and lower limbs. Patient was alert, oriented to time, place and person. He had experienced visual illusions more at night but not DT's. Physical exam disclosed mild finger tremors, diaphoresis, hepatomegaly, intense contraction, tonico-distal (carpal-pedal) in four limbs, painful palpation of contractions. No edema. Pinpoint sensation diminished and fasciculations more evident in both palms. With the Trousseau's maneuver and hyperventilation, the contractions got worse as well as distal numbness. Laboratory results were positive for hypocalcemia and hypomagnesemia 5 mg and 1.8 mgs (normal 5.9-6.6 and 2-4 mgs respectively). Muscle enzymes negative as well as urine. The above syndrome was rapidly resolved with the intravenous administration of magnesium sulfate 50 percent. The final diagnoses were alcoholic tetany/alcohol dependence/mixed depression-anxiety syndrome. The differential diagnoses with alcoholic polineuropathy/ alcoholic myopathy/hyperventilation syndrome/ idiopathic paroxistic myoglubinuria were ruled out.

I believe this syndrome is an example of altitude pathology because it is not found below thirteen thousand feet above sea level. Because it is frequently in La Paz. It has not been further studied; more evidence-based research needed. Due to its common presentation, it was never reported in the medical literature!

Etiology, Genetics, Neurochemistry, and Clinical Aspects

Etiology and Genetics

Three types of studies have conclusively proven the heredity of this disorder: family studies, identical twin studies, and adopted twin ones. One fascinating fact is that on one hand, some people are protected from becoming alcoholics ("the Oriental Flush Syndrome"), and on the other hand, people who using a colloquial saying "may drink somebody else under the table" are high risk to develop alcohol addiction. One pioneer of these studies in the USA is Mark Schuckit, MD. (34) Some take-home messages from Dr. Schuckit's research studies are the following:

- Alcohol addiction is influenced by genetics. When treating patients with alcoholism, look for opportunities to educate family about genetic influence. If it runs in your family, try not to drink.
- Alcoholism has many causes, but none relate to deficiency in morality. Studies of genes and environment allow identification of individuals at increased risk for alcoholism before they have begun drinking; information from environment provides basis of programs for preventing alcoholism. These studies are analogous to that for heart attacks (different genes that may predispose alcohol-metabolizing-enzyme mutations), high levels of impulsivity as seen in conduct disorder, and schizophrenia (increase overall risk for addictions).
- Mutations ALDH (alcohol dehydrogenase) is the enzyme that metabolizes alcohol to acetaldehyde and acetic acid. These mutations occur in individuals of Japanese, Chinese, and Korean ancestry. Because alcohol dehydrogenase produces acetaldehyde, those individuals' homozygous (they have the same two alleles) for gene accumulate acetaldehyde in blood, and the individual "becomes terribly sick" (similar to disulfiram-antabuse reaction that block the enzyme ALDH, and acetaldehyde accumulates). Those heterozygous for gene get red in the face, and heart rate increases; however they do not

tend to get sick. Generally, they should drink less than people who do not have mutations. In this sense, genetics protects them from becoming alcoholics.

Schuckit designed the San Diego Prospective Study. In 1978, he recruited 453 men twenty years of age. (50 percent were sons of alcoholics, and 50 percent were sons of controls with no alcoholism in the family. Daughters were studied separately; as participants were married, they totaled 370 together with their spouses. As they had children, they totaled 630 together with their children.) Participants were tested with several assessments: measurements of change in brain waves and hormone levels associated with alcohol consumption, survey of subjective feelings of intoxication, tests of motor performance, functional magnetic resonance imaging (MRI), swaying test for sensitivity to alcohol. All were also seen for follow-up every five years to determine how many developed alcoholism. Forty percent of children of alcoholics were less responsive at a given alcohol level than children of nonalcoholics.

- Heritability is explained by genes; 40 percent to 60 percent of level of response to alcohol are genetically influenced. Dr. Schuckit hopes to be able to identify (in adolescents) genotypes that increased risk of developing alcoholism; longitudinal studies (already thirty-five years of ongoing study) should determine which environmental interventions are most effective at a particular age in diminishing the influence of genes. However, it is impossible to totally prevent alcoholism. Nevertheless, the greater the understanding of risk factors, genes associated with them, and mechanisms through which they work, the better the chances for early identification and prevention. No small merit!

The etiology of alcoholism is multifactorial. The biopsychosocial model is the par excellence model necessary to understand it. However, the importance of genetics and neurochemistry deserves some considerations.

Neurochemistry and Clinical Aspects

Pharmacokinetics: What the Chemical Does to the Body

Alcohol is a water soluble molecule that is rapidly absorbed from the stomach into the bloodstream. Once in it, alcohol is rapidly distributed and gains access to all tissues, including the fetus in a pregnant women. The relationship between alcohol intake and blood level is body-weight dependent. Gender also contributes to it. When body weights are the same, women show a 20-25 percent higher blood alcohol level than men after ingesting the same amount of alcohol. This is due to less gastric metabolism of alcohol in women.

Alcohol is metabolized primarily by enzymatic pathways; only small amounts are excreted through the lungs as vapor. In the liver, alcohol is broken down by alcohol dehydrogenase (ADH), which converts alcohol into acetaldehyde, which consequently can be converted to acetate by the actions of acetaldehyde dehydrogenase (ALDH).

The rate of alcohol metabolism is relatively constant as the enzyme is saturated at relatively low blood alcohol levels. Alcohol metabolism averages approximately 1 ounce of pure alcohol per 3 hours in adults. Although stimulants are used to mask the depressant effects of alcohol, there do not appear to be any truly effective "alcohol antagonists" (amethystic agents). In most states in the USA, 0.5 mg of alcohol per 100 ml of blood is the legal limit. Figures above this number qualify for a DUI (driving under the influence).

Molecular Sites of Alcohol Action

Alcohol interacts with a variety of targets including both lipids and proteins. Alcohol's depressant action on neuronal excitability likely results from its ability to enhance the function of inhibitory ion channels while blocking the activity of excitatory receptors. The demonstration of effects on lipid-free systems have led to the idea that alcohol's actions are likely due to effects on ion channel proteins that regulate the excitability of the neuron. (35) The mechanism underlying the sensitivity of GABA (gamma-aminobutyric acid) release to alcohol is not currently known but could involve specific signaling pathways and proteins that normally regulate vesicle movement and fusion.

Glutamate is the major excitatory neurotransmitter and activates the ion channels called NMDA (N-methyl-D-aspartate) receptors. Alcohol has an antagonism of NMDA, which is involved in its rewarding properties because NMDA receptors are important in the regulation and release of dopamine in the nucleus accumbens. In this sense, it is similar to ketamine, which by a single intravenous infusion has been recently reported as rapidly improving treatment-resistant bipolar depression and suicidal ideation. Although other studies suggest that the enhancement of NMDA receptors after chronic alcohol may involve changes in the expression pattern of specific NMDA receptor subunits. (36)

Figure 4
Pleasure Centers of the Brain
NA: Nucleus Accumbens

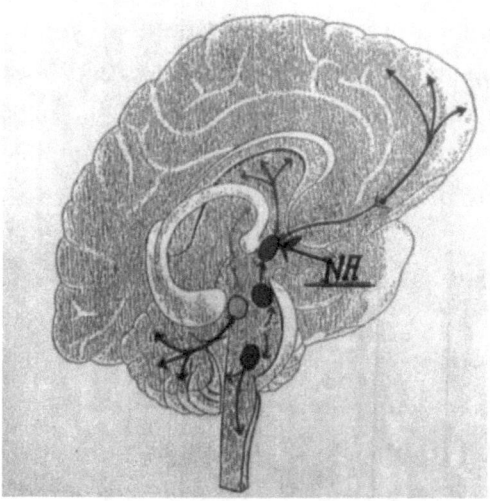

The <u>nucleus accumbens</u> is part of the pleasure centers of the brain. Originally described by Olds in 1954 (37) (Figure 4), which I think represents the anatomical locus of addictions, in general, and alcoholism, in particular, as well as the comorbidities with schizophrenia, bipolar disorders, anxiety/depressive disorders and OCD, and others. This nucleus is strategically located between the limbic system frontal cortex and the striatum. It is very rich in neurotransmitters such as dopamine, serotonin, endorphins. It is divided in a cortical and central zones. The central zone is more connected with the striatum and psychomotor disorders. Whereas the cortical zone is closely related to the olfactory system, the amygdala is very rich in dopaminergic receptors (clozapine has affinity for the receptor D4. Thus explaining why some patients on clozapine can diminish smoking) as well as opioid ones, which in turn are connected with serotonin receptors in the ventral tegmentum. The opioid receptors' deltas are stimulated by alcohol, which causes the release of dopamine in the nucleus accumbens causing alcohol craving. This may be one of the explanations why opiate blockers such as ReVia (naltrexone) may also diminish alcohol craving. Again because of the strategic location of the <u>nucleus accumbens</u>, it has a crucial role in the orchestration of many neurotransmitters released by addictive substances. It is important to remember that alcohol does not have affinity for any specific receptor but affects the molecular proteins such as the GABA and more the NMDA, which may also explain why medications such as acamprosate (Campral) that affect this receptor have antialcohol craving effects. To illustrate how little we know about how genetic factors affect alcohol drinking. Let's remember that among women we know even less. The prevalence of alcoholism among identical women twins is 31.6 percent. (38) Less than in men. It is possible that environmental factors play a more important role among women. The machismo factor tends to confirm this finding. However, and again to illustrate the complexity of interaction between genetic, gender, and ethnic factors, a higher prevalence of alcoholism among American Indian women was found. (39) Another study done by German scientists points out that at the anterior cingulate cortex during alcohol withdrawal in alcohol-dependent rodents, (40) the ratio of glutamate to glutamine rises sharply. It may prove useful as a biomarker for severity of alcohol dependence. It also corroborates why Acamprosate, considered an antiglutaminergic compound, is effective in some forms of alcoholism.

Types of Alcoholism

It was E. M. Jellineck who described four different types of alcoholism, which he divided with Greek letters. (41) They also indicate the progression of alcoholism. For historical reasons, I will briefly describe these four types: alpha, beta, gamma, delta alcoholism

- Alpha alcoholism is pure psychological, to relieve from emotional pain. It causes interpersonal problems, not real withdrawal or progression. It is also called "problem drinking."
- Beta alcoholism. We have medical complications such as polyneuropathy, gastritis, cirrhosis without psychological or physiological dependence. Social pressures and poor nutrition contribute to it.
- Gamma alcoholism. Tolerance to alcohol is developed; withdrawal and craving are present as well as loss of control. We observe the most severe damage. It is the most common type of alcoholism in the USA.
- Delta alcoholism. You add to gamma the inability to abstain from alcohol. Daily drinking frequently occurs. This would be the more severe type of alcoholism. This classification is not so practical. I prefer the division between type I and II proposed by Cloninger et al. and the type A and B proposed by Babor. (42)

Type I and A share the following:

- Later onset of alcoholism after the age of twenty-five
- Fewer childhood behavior problems
- Mild alcohol-related problems and fewer hospitalizations

- Lower degree of novelty seeking and preference toward harm avoidance

Type II and B are almost the opposite of type I and A:

- Familial alcoholism
- Earlier onset of alcohol-related problems before age 25
- More severe alcohol-related problems and violence
- Preference for risk taking or novelty seeking behavior

Another more recent classification of alcoholism and comorbidity suggests four types:

- Alcoholism and depression/anxiety disorders
- Alcoholism, schizophrenia, and bipolar disorders
- Alcoholism and personality disorders such as antisocial
- Alcoholism and AIDS

Regarding the use of medications, many patients, especially Latinos, are refractory to monotherapy requiring careful polypharmacy to diminish alcohol craving with antidepressants, second generation antipsychotics, such as clozapine (Clozaril), risperidone (Risperdal), olanzepine (Zyprexa), quetiapine (Seroquel), ziprasidone (Geodon), lurasidone (Latuda), iloperidone (Fanapt), asenapin (Saphris), and other mood stabilizer such as, carbamazepine (Tegretol), lamotrigine (Lamictal) or valproic acid (Depakote). The latter, and according to Shalloum, has an anti-alcohol-craving effect.

In alcoholism, according Dr. Willenbring, (43) in the next decade, "development of more effective pharmaceuticals and identification of indicators predicting response in individual patients will be central features. Having more effective, cost-effective, and appealing treatments and driven to system changes to facilitate their implementation." At present, most treatment offered lasts a few weeks for a disorder that last years. Let's remember that 40 percent of daily or nearly daily heavy drinkers meet the criteria for alcohol addiction. Along the same lines, only 20 to 40 percent of individuals with alcoholic liver cirrhosis also have alcohol addiction. About the fascinating field of alcoholism, there is still so much to be learned.

However, nothing replaces the importance of AA as explained above. Patients who attend AA meetings for two years may be totally abstinent in 80 percent of cases. This is an example of the empowerment that having group therapy (AA) and possibly making astral connections can have in the rehabilitation of alcoholism.

Among physicians addicted to alcohol most of them recover. Their treatment is sort of unique; they have a very strong motivation to keep their medical license active! They are closely monitored, and in many cases, they have "hit bottom"; they are coerced in some way and sicker when they enter in treatment. They may have more social dysfunction, more medical consequences, or are simply more complicated to treat. For instance, in a study of 100 doctors addicted to alcohol followed for twenty-one years, 73 percent had recovered (44).

COCAINE ADDICTION

As not two faces, so no two cases are alike in all respects, and unfortunately is not only the disease itself which is so varied, but the subjects themselves have peculiarities which modify its action.
—Sir William Osler, *Teaching and Thinking*

History

The history of cocaine addiction is very much related to the history of the coca plant. Indigenous to Bolivia and Peru, cocaine is one of the fourteen alkaloids isolated from the coca leaves by the Viennese chemist Alfred Niemann in 1859 (45).

Figure 5

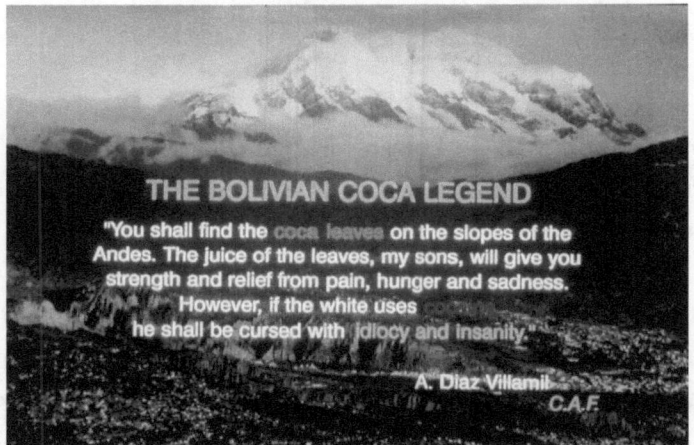

THE BOLIVIAN COCA LEGEND

"You shall find the coca leaves on the slopes of the Andes. The juice of the leaves, my sons, will give you strength and relief from pain, hunger and sadness. However, if the white uses he shall be cursed with idiocy and insanity."

A. Diaz Villamil
C.A.F.

I would like to start quoting a Bolivian writer Diaz Villamil (46) who wrote *The Bolivian Coca Legend (Figure 5)*, and because as the saying goes, "A picture is worth a thousand words." I hope we learned from it.

This legend predicted the devastating effects of cocaine in the Western world. The legend conveys the message that should help us understand coca chewing as a cultural tradition and perhaps some positive effects for the Peru-Bolivian Indians.

Figure 6
Trephination Among the Peru-Bolivian Indians
(Courtesy of Parke Davis)

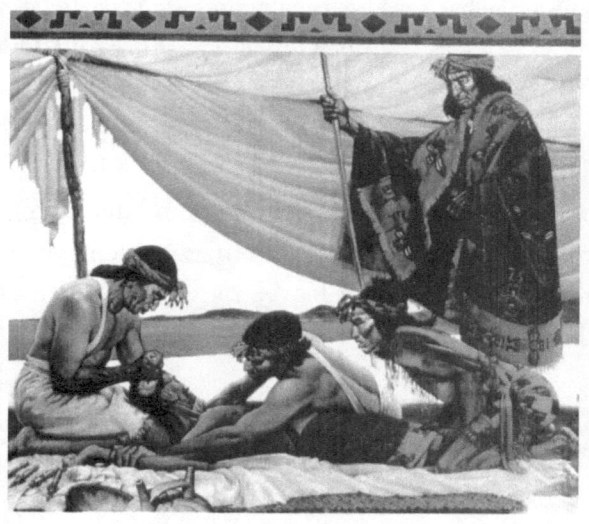

However, the Indians have known for centuries about the only medical use of cocaine as a local anesthetic. This is the only recognized medical and scientific use of cocaine.

What is not very well known is that trepanation was still being performed by the Aymara Indians from Bolivia (Figure 6) until the end of the nineteenth century as reported by A. F. Bandelier (47). Bandelier had been investigating Indian ruins in Bolivia for the American Museum of Natural History of New

York. He spent a great part of 1895 on Lake Titicaca and its shores. He found sixty-five trephining crania out of 1,200. Bandelier reported that trephining was done by the Aymara medicine men called *kolliris* for mystical reasons against diseases attributed to spiritual influences, such as chronic headaches. Bandelier refers to the anesthetic properties of coca as follows: "The Indians have no anesthetics, properly so called, but the constant use (or I might say abuse) of coca creates insensibility. The plant is always applied by them to wounds, bruises, and contusions, and it certainly tends to deaden the pain, if not eliminate it. In this manner, the Indians unconsciously employ an anesthetic, although they believe only in its healing qualities." No doubt that coca chewing and cocaine addiction are the opposite sides of the same coin illustrated in the Bolivian coca legend (Figure 5).

Coca chewing and cocaine addiction are separate sides of the same coin: cocaine. In order to understand these two ironic aspects of cocaine, the biopsychosocial model must be applied. However, with the tragic Mexican war on drugs, according Alvaro Riveros Tejada, (48) "the governments of Chile, Brazil, and the Catholic Church have expressed their serious concern to the Bolivian government, regarding the transformation of the sacred leaves into a criminal matter. Cocaine has been converted in 'Coca nostra'."

Figure 7

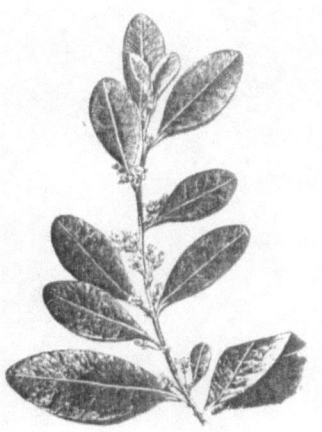

Bolivian Coca Leaves

Along these lines, I will describe a very important contribution that help us understand the importance of coca chewing for the Indians. Written by an American and a Bolivian, Carter and Mamani (49-50) as well as refer the reader to the classical Sigmund Freud paper "Uber Coca" (51-52). In the latter, Freud describes accurately the coca plant and plantations(Figures:7-7b); he also describes seven therapeutic cocaine applications, ironically only the last one being accurate: its local anesthetic property. "No doubt the local anesthetic properties of cocaine will have important future applications." He let escape through his fingers the opportunity of becoming famous. This was reserved for Dr. Koller. However, Freud correctly described cocaine as an stimulant. He made the mistake of personally using, recommending it for the treatment of alcoholism and cocainism. He was attacked by Erlenmeyer and Louis Lewin who stated, "It becomes a dual addiction." As a result of these attacks, he declined his studies on cocaine and dedicated himself to the establishment of psychoanalysis. From the historical point of view, not a small merit!

Figure 7b
Coca Plantations "Cocales" in Yungas, Bolivia

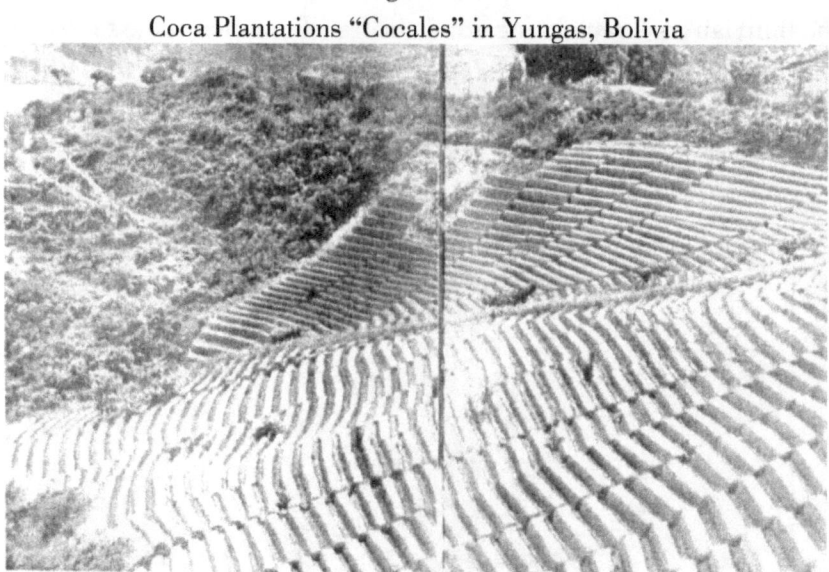

Dr. Kurt Koller, (53) an ophthalmologist, a contemporary of Freud, by serendipity, discover this property: "On one occasion, Dr. Engel and I compared notes experimenting with cocaine. Engel stated 'how it numbs the tongue,' and Koller answered, 'Yes, everyone who has tried it by mouth has noted the same.' That moment I realized I had in my pocket the medication I was trying to discover for years." His successful experiments led to the scientific discovery that cocaine is an excellent ophthalmological local anesthetic that he used for ophthalmological surgery. His official presentation was given at the International Society of Ophthalmology in Heidelberg on September 15, 1884. He was declared a "Benefactor of Humanity." The fact was that the Aymara Bolivian Indians knew it for four thousand years!

Carter and Mamani—their very valuable book, but not so popular because as far as I know it has not been translated into the English language since it was published in Spanish in 1984 when the destructive effects of cocaine addiction were in its apex especially in this country. This book explains to the Westerner the importance for adaptation and survival; it has nothing to say from the sociological spiritual and astral value of this plant. In Bolivia, they carried on a very important survey, the only one in its nature. Let me remind the reader that their experiments were with coca chewing not cocaine addiction. Their survey was conducted among 2,712 farmers and 277 miners. The prevalence of *acullicu* (coca chewing) was 82 percent among farmers and 88 percent among miners.

To the question put to them, "Why do you chew coca leaves?" 81 percent stated it was for working (this was very ingeniously used by the Spaniards conquistadors to exploit the richest silver mountain in the world, the Potosí Mountain), 78 percent for medicine, 63 percent against hunger, 55 percent to stay awake, 55 percent to socialize, and 44 percent to tell fortune. One important aspect is its antidepressant effects. Orphans and widows answered, "Due to sadness, I use coca." Nothing to say about the social peer pressure. On the mental health aspects. Among miners, they use coca for "El Tio," the imaginary god-owner of the richest portions of a mine. Chewing coca, they have better self-confidence and optimism against the fear of mining in obscures mine corridors. It is also useful to protect them against landslides in the mines. At age 15, the young Aymaras are sent by their parents away from home with "the protection of the sacred leaves of the race, their leaves will protect them against, hunger, cold, pain, and all kinds of sufferings."

Coca chewing in Bolivia is called *acullicu,* which is in the Quechua language the most popular name. It also means a 5' rest, similar to our coffee break or the Russian *perekur* (In the Russian language means smoking break), and the persons engaged in it are called *acullicadores.* In the Aymara language, it is called *pijchar*; in Peru, it is called *chajchar.* The European perception, due to their ignorance of the Indian culture, is in general mistaken and negative. In the Westerner culture, the real world is separated from the supernatural or astral. For the Quechua and Aymara Indians, both worlds overlap. It seems that from the historical point of view, the first European who described it was Amerigo Vespucci who mistakenly thought the Indians were chewing tobacco.

In Bolivia, in many hotels, the coca leaves are presented to tourists for their treatment of "altitude sickness," in the form of tea or mixed with baking soda. The amount of cocaine extracted may be about 0.5-1.5 mg. of cocaine. The coca-chewing person selects carefully the leaves for a more bitter taste, which have more cocaine. As the social drinker drinks slowly and lower amounts of alcohol, the *acullicadores* do the same.

In summary, Carter-Mamani's book are against *coca eradication* (remember their study was in the late seventies). They postulate that it will be like violating human rights: "the millenary tradition has thought the Peru-Bolivian Indians how to use the coca alkaloids in a constructive way. Nowadays when the international politics are all about human rights, not to allow the descendants of the first inhabitants of the Americas to recognize their rights would be inadmissible . . . All over the world there is no drug that gets close to coca. This is a unique phenomenon indigenous only to Peru-Bolivian Indians. To understand it and establish an adequate and humane political climate constitutes one of the most important challenges of the 20th (and 21st) century."

Figure 8

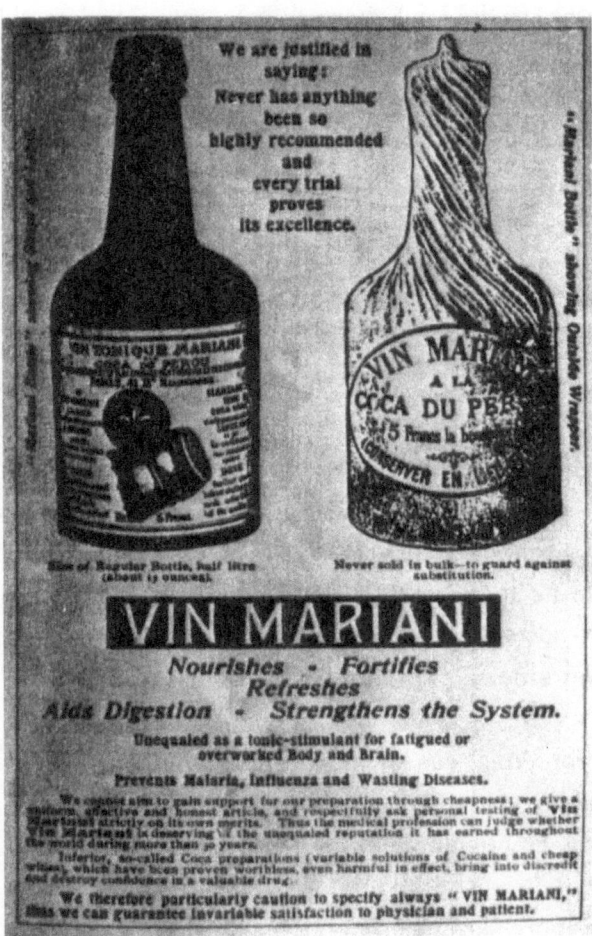

The 1980s' cocaine epidemic was the third epidemic in this country. The first epidemic started in 1880s. Apparently, it was begun by an Italian neurologist Paolo Mantegazza (54) who lived in Peru, telling very compelling and inspiring comments, such as "I prefer to live only ten years full of coca instead of a million of centuries without it," then another Italian Angelo Mariani, a chemist in Corcega. He apparently was the first one to import cocaine to Europe and made a very famous wine with it. He called it Vin Mariani (Figure 8). It was considered a panacea. He wrote thirteen books about his wine and was endorsed by important contemporary luminaries such as the Pope Leo XIII, Anatole France, H. G. Welss Thomas Edison, and Jules Verne. In the USA, immediately, it was endorsed by many, and many products containing cocaine were manufactured and sold. Even the English tea was attempted to be replaced by coca tea. In Philadelphia, cigarettes of coca were made (55).

The next famous product containing cocaine was Coca-Cola, introduced in 1886 by an Atlanta chemist, John Stith Pemberton. Coca-Cola was also endorsed as a panacea including its use against depression! Two years later, the new owner, Asa G. Chandler, promoted Coca-Cola as a refreshment drink, which continued to contain cocaine until 1903. Since then, many transformations of the Coca-Cola bottle have been seen. The last one on December 1, 2011 (56) when "Coca-Cola abandons the white can" due to its confusion with Diet Coca-Cola. Let me remind the reader that this was the second legal import of cocaine, the other one as local anesthetic. Its promotion continued probably until 1914 with the introduction of the "Harrison Narcotic Act." It was forbidden ever since.

The second epidemic was in the twenties; it was a transient epidemic restricted mainly to the use of bohemians and musicians. Then it was replaced by the amphetamines.

The third and more serious epidemic took place in the eighties. We have learned something from the last cocaine epidemic of the 1980s. However, until now, we do not have a medication for the specific treatment of cocaine addiction. We have off-label medications such as amantadine, baclofen, buprenorphine, Inderal, and topiramate and the research on a vaccine.

Neurochemistry

The neurochemical explanation of addictions can be illustrated with Nora Volkov's explanation using MRI (Magnetic Resonant Imaging) of cocaine addiction. This explanation is found in chapter 1 of *Principles of Addiction Medicine, Fourth Edition*, "Drug Addiction: The Neurobiology of Behavior Gone Awry."(57) She has been working for more than thirty years with MRI in addicted persons. She has proven that these persons have an "anatomic locus" for their addiction. Not a small merit!

It is the case that addicted persons are born with a deficiency in certain neurotransmitters and that they try to self-medicate usually with the wrong chemical! If we can replace this deficiency (that is what buprenorphine does with opiates), then they function normally!

Obviously, persons addicted to cocaine are not criminals, and jails are the wrong place for them. They have to be medically treated.

Dr. Nora Volkov's (who happens to be the great-granddaughter of Leon Trotsky) work has been pointed out as a crucial one by Dr. Alan Leshner, (58) who in 1997, when he was the director of NIDA (National Institute of Drug Abuse), published a seminal article "Addiction Is a Brain Disease, and It Matters," which is summarized as follows.

The pleasure center of the brain, which was discovered by Olds (37) in 1954 is the anatomical locus of addictions (Figure 4). It is located in the limbic system. The ventral tegmentum, nucleous accumbens, with projections to the frontal lobes. However this simple anatomical description is a bit more complicated.

Her explanation about the anatomical locus of addiction was presented while talking about cocaine dependence but very well can be applied to other addictions. Let's remember, to understand addictions, a biopsychosocial model is needed. From the biological component. Dr.

Volkov's (now the director of NIDA) work with PET (positron emission tomography) scans in persons addicted to cocaine for over thirty years has proven the following: "imaging studies have documented that disrupted dopamine activity in the brain (shown by reductions in dopamine D2 receptors) is associated with abnormal activity in the orbitofrontal cortex (OFC) and in the anterior cingulate gyrus brain regions that are involved in salience attribution and inhibitory control." Their disruption is linked to compulsive behavior, OCD (obsessive-compulsive disorder). Dr. Volkov's last lecture at the APA (American Psychiatric Association) in Honolulu emphasizes the importance of the integrated treatment of comorbidity (59). The abnormalities in these cortical regions could underlie the compulsive nature of drug administration and their inability to control their intake. At the cellular level, drugs have been reported to alter the expression of certain transcription factors (regulating their transcription into mRNA) and numerous other proteins in brain regions that are regulated by dopamine. At the circuit level, there is clear evidence that adaptations in the mesocortical circuit cause compulsive drug administration, and they probably participate in relapse. Adaptations also seems to occur in the mesolimbic circuit (including the nucleus accumbens, amygdala, and hippocampus), which probably cause the enhanced saliency or important value of the drug. Adaptations have also been reported in the nigrocortical circuit (including the dorsal striatum), which might underlie habits, also the curious prevalence of comorbidity, OCD among the anxiety disorders, and other mood disorders.

Genetic Factors

It is estimated that 40-60 percent of the vulnerability to addiction is due to genetic factors. In humans, several chromosomal regions have been linked to drug abuse, but only a few genes have been identified with polymorphisms (alleles) that either protect or predispose to addiction. For example, specific alleles for the genes that encode alcohol dehydrogenases ADH1B and ALDH2 are reportedly protective against alcoholism (they are responsible for the "flush reaction to alcohol" explained above). D2 receptor polymorphisms have been linked to a higher vulnerability to drug addiction. However, its replication is still pending.

Comorbidity with Mental Illness

The high prevalence of smoking that is initiated after individuals experience depression could reflect, in part, the antidepressant effects of nicotine as well as the antidepressant effects of monoamine oxidase A and B inhibition by cigarette smoke. This highlights the importance of early evaluation and treatment of mental disorders as an effective strategy to prevent drug addiction that starts as self-medication: giving the patients the proper antidepressant medication.

Preventing Addiction

The greater vulnerability of adolescents to experimentation with drugs of abuse and to subsequent addiction underscores why prevention of early exposure is such an important strategy to combat drug addiction. Tailored interventions that take into account socioeconomic, cultural, age, and gender characteristics of children and adolescents are more likely to improve the effectiveness of the interventions. In the future, as we gain knowledge of the genes and proteins that they encode and that make a person more or less vulnerable to addiction, more targets will be available to tailored interventions for those at high risk.

What separates the Peru-Bolivian Indians who chew coca leaves from the addicted person? Let me clarify that this does not mean that there are no Indians who are addicted to coca-leaves chewing, not too many in my experience. If they lose control, have a compulsive use of it, and they do it despite negative biopsychosocial consequences, they are addicted. Coca-leaves chewing may have served a social purpose when the conquistadores exploited Indians to extract silver from the famous mountain, Potosi. They may continue using it under controlled conditions.

However, epidemiological studies are missing. In any case, the answer is a biopsychosocial one, especially genetic.

Clinical Aspects

With smokable cocaine dubbed "crack" in the USA, its production is simple: the cocaine hydrochloride is dissolved in water. To make the solution alkaline, baking soda is added. The mixture is heated to eliminate water. The result is crack. Its name came from the noise on the cracks of the walls were it is produced. It costs about $10 per rock of crack. This form of smokable cocaine is also called freebasing; it apparently started in the Bahamas where in the eighties an increase in the admissions due to their addiction at the only psychiatric hospital, Sandilands Rehabilitation Hospital, in New Providence was noted. The number went from none in 1982 to 60 in 1983 and 523 in 1984. A paper published in Lancet constitutes the first report due to almost exclusively freebasing cocaine. Then it spread to Los Angeles and the rest of the country.

From a historical, chronological, and geographic point of view, it was in Bolivia and Peru where the first reports of smoking cocaine came from. In Bolivia, a pioneering research paper was published by two psychiatrists, one of them our friend and colleague Dr. Nils Noya. (60) They noted in San Pedro, La Paz prison that all the patients reported that once they began to smoke, they could not stop until all the supplies were consumed. A withdrawal syndrome, the first one, (1979) was reported as a depressive rebound syndrome. The Bolivian psychiatrist stated, "However, the main symptoms of intoxication disappeared, showing the patients inverse phenomena, such as slowness in thought, depressive mood, asthenia, adynamia, anhedonia, and suicidality."

Another early report comes from F. Jeri, MD, (61) of Lima, Peru. Dr. Jeri studied 188 patients who were treated because of severe compulsive cocaine smoking. The severity of this addiction and the recalcitrant response to standard treatments required in Peru bold interventions such as bilateral cingulotomies. Needless to say, these efforts, which are ethically questionable, and as far as I know, have not been successful and must take no place in the twenty-first century.

The most common cocaine medical complications that we often see are listed below:

- From snorting (intranasal): rhinitis sinusitis, ethmoiditis, anosmia, epistaxis, and perforated nasal septum (almost pathognomonic of cocaine snorting)
- From shooting up (intravenous needle tracks): AIDS, hepatitis, endocarditis, vasculopaties, sepsis, meningitis, abscesses
- From smoking: COPD, alveolar rupture, pneumothorax, bloody expectorate, backache, shoulder pain (posture-related), burns, madarosis (loss of eyelashes), sudden death (hyperpyrexia), cerebral hemorrhage (acute hypertension), rupture of ascending aorta, intestinal ischemia
- MI among young patients due to vasospasm of coronary artery, increased blood pressure, increased demand for oxygen
- Seizures "kindling," status epilepticus
- Respiratory arrest (inhibition of medullary center in the midbrain), "body packers," overdose (OD)
- Cardiac arrhythmia, ventricular fibrillation
- OD due to congenital pseudocholinesterase deficiency

Psychiatric

- Manic behavior: euphoria, hyper alertness, paranoia, violent, homicidal behavior
- Anhedonia, anergia, anorexia, severe depression, suicidal ideation and planning.
- Misperceptions: hallucinations ("coke bugs"), psychosis
- Panic attacks, insomnia, irritability

- Polydrug dependence: marijuana-cocaine/opioids-cocaine/ alcohol-cocaine (the production of coca-ethylene may be lethal), nicotine-cocaine

Other

- Unexplained weight loss, malnutrition, and hypovitaminosis
- Sexual dysfunctions
- Obstetrical: increased spontaneous abortion; "Cocaine babies" with congenital malformations and neurobehavioral impairments
- Bruxism and dental disorders
- Others

The crack epidemic in the eighties have taught us the many medical/ psychiatric complications often found with cocaine. Criminal and violent behavior related to cocaine craving, cocaine-induced paranoid syndrome, and a severe depressive syndrome perhaps due to kindling mechanisms (reverse tolerance in the limbic system).

OPIOID ADDICTION

Current medications are given with more skill. We know better their indications and contraindications. We can tell with certainty that due to a mistake in dosage, hundreds improve.
—Sir William Osler, *Pills and Poisons*

History

Opioid OD quadrupled in 2008 over the last decade 4.8/100.000 for opioids compared with just 2.8/100.000 for illicit drugs, including heroin, cocaine, hallucinogens, or stimulants. According to a report from the Centers for Disease Control and Prevention (62) by 2008 OD reached 36,450 deaths almost as many as from motor vehicle crashes (39,973). Opioid pain reliever (OPRs) sales have also increased with the OD rate in 2008 nearly four times the rate in 1999. The substance abuse treatment admission rate in 2009 was almost six times the rate in 1999. "By 2010, enough OPRs were sold each year to medicate every American adult with 5 mg of hydrocodone every four hours for one month," the researches said.

Opioids are drugs derived from the poppy seed. The term *narcotics* is confusing. It is used to include all drugs that require control by the DEA (Drug Enforcement Administration) especially the ones that cause analgesia and stupor. The word *opos* comes from the Greek (in Latin *opium*) and means "juice." In antiquity, it was a symbol of "eternal sleep." Its popularity increased with the father of chemistry Paracelsus, who recognized its value to relieve pain and depression as well as the treatment of insomnia and many other ailments. One of the most common therapeutic formulas was called Laudanum (from the Latin for something "commendable"). Like most of the addictive drugs, at small dosages, it has therapeutic value; besides once it is taken orally, the first metabolic passage in the liver helps its metabolism and detoxification. However, smoking opium or using it IV (intravenous) the value of dosage is multiplied and causes toxicity and death due to respiratory depression. This is why opium put almost the whole Chinese nation in a complete stupor, allowing England to win the "opium wars." This problem was resolved by Mao Tse-Tung, who with a stroke of his pen, at the beginning of the sixties, declared it to be totally forbidden.

The history of the treatment of opioids is long and always changing. One must be especially careful in recommending new techniques that should meet the two demands of safety and efficacy. Kolb and Himmelsbach (1938) looked back on forty years of almost futile attempts to treat it.Including "Cold Turkey." Portrayed in the movie *The Man with the Golden Arm* with Frank Sinatra. No one who is young and in fair physical health dies from it. However, because the withdrawal from opioids "is a bitch," very unpleasant, it leads many to self-medicate again with opioids, and the vicious cycle is established. Having buprenorphine available, there is no need to "cold-turkey" detoxification. Just the opposite happens with alcohol and other sedatives. Their withdrawal can be life-threatening. I will make the point that detoxification is not the treatment of addictions but a Band-Aid solution!

Going back to the birth of Addiction Medicine in America (1750-1935)

Before Benjamin Rush, in 1774, the philanthropist Anthony Benezet (63) published "Mighty Destroyer Displayed." Alcohol was described as "bewitching poison." He noted the existence of "unhappy dram-drinkers bound in slavery" with the tendency of drunkenness to self-accelerate (loss of control) Drops begets drams, and drams begets more drams, till they became to be without weight or measure." Benezet's warnings were followed by Dr. B. Rush's (1746-1813) publication of his 1874 book *Inquiry into the Effects of Ardent Spirits on the Human Body and Mind* (24). It was the first treatise on alcoholism. Rush was the first physician in the USA to state that many persons addicted to alcohol could be restored to full health and responsible citizenship with the creation of a special facility (a "sober house") to care for them. American physicians specializing in addiction began publishing texts on the nature of addiction and their treatment methods, such as *Drugs That Enslave: The Opium, Morphine, Chloral, and Hashish Habits*, which was published in the 1860s by Dr. H. H. Cane; Dr. Fred Hubbard's *The Opium Habit and Alcoholism*. The central concept was that of "inebriate," viewed as a disease. These addictions were meticulously detailed by clinical subpopulation and drug choice. The growing field of addiction medicine was infused with optimism in the early 1890s. Dr. Hubbard stated, "The future looks promising, and it is believed that the public will support inebriate asylums with increasing generosity." However, forces outside the medical profession would drive a knife between the physician and those persons addicted to drugs and alcohol.

Demedicalization and the Collapse of Addiction Treatment (1900-1935)

Regarding the opioid addiction in America, I follow Dr. Renner's article written in the Handbook of Office-Based Buprenorphine Treatment of Opioid Dependence, "Opioid Dependence in America" (64). It traces the evolution of "opioid addiction" (as I prefer to call it) from the era of opium-laced patent medicines, through injection of morphine after the Civil War, to the heroin epidemics of the twentieth century, and finally the opioid "pharmaceutical abuse," as Dr. Renner calls it, that began in the 1990s. It concludes, "The introduction of office-based buprenorphine treatment is best understood as an effort to restore a medical treatment model and a more coherent public health approach to what has become an intractable medical, legal, and social problem."

Nonetheless the technological advances of the nineteenth century led to the isolation of morphine. Its commercial distribution began in 1832. In addition, the hypodermic syringe was invented, which allowed the intramuscular use of morphine a more effective way to treat combat injuries after the Civil War. It became a common medical practice for physicians to give morphine as a long-term treatment to treat chronic pain, which by the way, is being resurrected today as new opioids are being marketed. Let me list them:

- In January 2011, the FDA approved Abstral (Prostrakan), a fentanyl transmucosal tablet indicated for the treatment of breakthrough cancer pain.
- Approved in 2010, Exalgo (Mallinckrodt) is an extended-release formulation of hydromorphone, indicated once-daily for moderate to severe pain. The formulation uses a new osmotic, controlled-release oral delivery system in which osmosis attracts water in the body to the inside of the capsule to trigger release of hydromorphone. It takes about six hours to get effective levels of hydromorphone; in 4-5 days, it reaches a steady state in the body.
- The FDA, also in 2010, approved buprenorphine patch (Butrans; Perdue-Pharma) in 5, 10, 20 mcg/hour doses for patients with moderate to severe pain requiring around-the-clock opioid treatment.
- Nucynta (tapentadol) in 50, 75, 100 mg is reported as safe and "no street value." This is not a long-acting opioid; it requires use every 4-7 hours.
- There are at least three more opioids in the pipeline. These opioids will require training on how to prescribe them. The FDA announced that it will require the sixteen prescription manufacturers that sell long-acting or extended-release opioids to provide education materials for physicians and patients regarding the risk of opioid drug use. The FDA plans a risk evaluation and mitigation

strategy (REMS) in place by early 2012. These measures came as a result of the increased number of Americans in 2009 aged 12 and older abusing pain relievers. It has increased 20 percent since 2002 from 29 million to 37 million. Furthermore in May 2011, as a recognition of the important role that physicians play in the prescription of opioids and in this epidemic (65), the key is "to balance benefits while mitigating risks is a key challenge to physicians and other prescribes and calls for targeted education and training to improve the screening and management of pain and the use of opioid medication."

The patient who is low risk of abusing opioids medication is someone who has the following:

- Presenting diagnosis is severe chronic pain syndrome, including cancer, not relieved by previous interventions.
- Negative history for addiction, personal and familial
- Negative history of comorbidities, psychiatric or medical

This leaves us with probably a minority of patients. The rest require the FDA REMS evaluation and a lot of education to see if the patient takes the medication as prescribed. This simple recommendation will decrease the number of person who became addicted to opioids. If this is the case, find out if your patient is the appropriate "optimal" patient for buprenorphine (see below) under clinical use issues.

To my knowledge, only a recent book *Responsible Opioid Prescription* (66) has been released, sponsored by the Federation of State Medical Boards. This little book is highly recommended but has no chapter devoted to buprenorphine. It spells out seven concise principles:

1. Evaluation of the patient
2. Treatment plan
3. Informed consent agreement for treatment

4. Periodic review
5. Referral and Patient Management
6. Documentation
7. Compliance with controlled substances laws and regulations as a solution for the dilemma of treating patients in pain and avoiding the opioid diversion "Pharmacovigilance."

Opioid overdose is now the second leading cause of unintentional death in the United States, second only to motor-vehicle crashes, prompting the CDC (Center for Diseases Control) to label pharmaceutical opioid overdose a national epidemic.

In the 1960s, a very important contribution to the treatment of opioid dependence was found. Methadone maintenance. It was Vincent Doyle, an internist at the Rockefeller Institute (now the Rockefeller University) with his wife, Mary Nyswander, a psychiatrist (67). In 1965, they published their landmark paper on the efficacy of this treatment. The legalization of methadone maintenance treatment occurred in 1972, which reversed the Harrison Act. This was a crucial event. Both stressed the importance of adequate methadone dose to block the euphoria caused by heroin, also the need for long-term if not indefinite treatment, and the importance of counseling and other support services. Over the next thirty years, there were rarely more than one hundred thousand addicts in methadone maintenance treatment, less than 10 percent of the population in need for this treatment. Despite of their evidence-based, demonstrated efficacy of treatment and the first drug that prevents AIDS among the patients who are on methadone maintenance! Not small merit in medicine. This was never welcomed by the majority of addicts or by most communities, plus the bad reputation that soon the methadone clinics received notice to explain its limitation.

I will briefly mention the most comprehensive review of the long-term course of opioid addiction. Hser et al. (68) conducted a thirty-three-year follow-up of 581 male heroin addicts treated in the California Civil Addict

Program from 1962 to 1997. 284 individuals (48 percent of the original sample) had died. Among the 242 survivors, 40.5 percent had used heroin within the past year. Also 22.1 percent were daily alcohol drinkers, and many others reported other illicit drug abuse. Only 22 percent were abstinent, and another 6 percent were in methadone maintenance treatment. Overall, this crucial study demonstrates the lethality of opioid addiction. Heroin addiction was demonstrated to be a chronic lifetime disorder with severe health and social consequences.

The New Epidemic of the Abuse of Pain Relievers

Why this epidemic? Maybe drug dealers are well informed about the new attitude to treat pain. They anticipated it, and here we are. What will the next epidemic be?

The introduction of Talwin in the 1960 caused a short period of abuse when it was discovered that injecting a combination of Talwin and amphetamines (T's and blues) produced a good euphoria. This problem was apparently resolved after the FDA ordered a reformulation of Talwin with naloxone (Talwin Nx). The abuse of opioids remained as a low problem until more potent pain medications were introduced with low abuse potential and longer duration of action. The formulation of morphine sulfate (MS Contin). In 1996, Perdue resolved the problem of adapting these features with the introduction of OxyContin, an acrylic formulation of oxycodone that dissolves slowly and provided about twelve hours of pain relief. Doses from 10 mg to 160 mg can be given. Perdue was permitted to market OxyContin, a first-line medication for the treatment of nonmalignant pain. Within 2-3 years of its introduction, doctors in rural Maine and Virginia reported that young people were crushing the tablets and injecting or snorting them. It also reflected the widespread use of illicit Percocet (oxycodone-acetaminophen) and Vicoden (hydrocodone-acetaminophen). By 2000, the number of abusers tripled to 2.5 million, and in 2007, 5.2 million of Americans—2.1 percent of individuals twelve and older—reported using prescription pain relievers for no-medical reasons in the past month. In 2007, there were 2,147,000 new initiates. The mean age of use for new initiates in 2007 was 21.2 years. This new breed of abusers tends to be younger, better educated, and less antisocial than the typical heroin addict. They use it mainly orally or by snorting it. They are also more likely to have psychiatric comorbidity such as depression and anxiety. It reminds us about self-medication. Of course, the danger with these medications is OD (overdose). Oxycodone pure contains 30 mg; it is called "Perc 30s" or "Roxies." Oxymorphone (Opama) is time release similar to OxyContin, and it is causing a rush of OD.

The fact that we have treated these patients as criminals is reason enough to change this false stereotype. Addicted patients have a brain disorder inherited in most cases. What they have been doing is self-medicating with the wrong chemical that in many cases can kill them. Not with buprenorphine alone. In this sense I believe is the best medication we have in addiction medicine. Nonetheless because many of these patients need limit-setting a biopsychosocial model is the par excellence model to be applied. This biopsychosocial triad is the emblem signified in the Celtic cross and many other occult and astral issues. As scientists and professionals in the medical field we should emphasize the scientific knowledge we have about addictions. Started with Olds and the pleasure center of the brain that has been much refined with the work of Dr. Norah Volkov.

Psychiatrists need to be well prepared if they opt to treat pain with opioids. Most psychiatrists do not prescribe opioids; it is outside the realm of our training. However, we know that patients who abuse substances have higher rates of chronic pain than that of those who do not abuse substances. Psychiatrists should prescribe timed-release opioids because patients are not going to have euphoria from them. Psychiatrists should be aware that procedural options exist to relieve pain and minimize its abuse in this at-risk population such as radiofrequency denervation, peripheral and spinal neurostimulation, as well as intrathecal infusion therapy, which can combine many nonopioid medications, such as local anesthetics, clonidine, and ziconotide with low doses of opioids if needed.

The challenge is to separate the different groups of patients addicted to opioids to prescribe the proper medication. For instance, who would benefit from naltrexone or methadone or buprenorphine? No doubt psychiatric pharmacogenomics will help (69). Meantime, we have to use our clinical acumen.

Buprenorphine and Neurochemistry

Buprenorphine prescription goes back to the year 2000 when their research was approved during President Clinton's administration and the Drug Addiction Treatment Act of 2000 (DATA). *Doctors who are licensed to prescribe buprenorphine can be found at SAMHSA Treatment Locator. com.* (Add underlined) Finally in October 2002, the prescription under schedule III of buprenorphine (two sublingual pill preparations: Suboxone/ Subutex) was FDA approved.

Buprenorphine and the Return to Office-Based Treatment

Two books are recommended to make yourself more familiar with buprenorphine. (70) and (64)

The first one, "the buprenorphine bible," was published in 2004. Its title: *Clinical Guidelines for the Use of Buprenorphine in the Treatment of Opioid Addiction* (70). A treatment improvement protocol (TIP 40) published by the US Department of Health and Human Services. This book contains six chapters and ten appendices with ten expert panel members. It is a very good reference book. The second one, *Handbook of Office-Based Buprenorphine Treatment of Opioid Dependence* written by Dr. J. A. Renner and P. Levounis, (64) is a nice update on buprenorphine. It was published in 2011. It has fourteen chapters and two appendices. It tells us what we have learned from buprenorphine after using it for eight years. However, I disagree with their excessive caution on the use of quetiapine; instead they should say "judicious use of quetiapine" because quetiapine is sedative it is used to help sleep and also as a mood stabilizer for patients with comorbid bipolar disorders. It has been abused by some. Any medication can be abused. That does not mean it is addictive. Its value in the treatment of comorbid bipolar disorder and depression is important. For addictive persons with comorbid bipolar disorder and when it is properly prescribed, this medication, quetiapine (Seroquel), especially the XR form, can be very useful. The history of opioid treatment in this country, according Dr. Rolley E. "Ed" Johnson, the vice president of Reckitt Benkiser, the manufacturer of Suboxone (71) has been alternating with attitudes of opening and closing the treatment door for our patients. Let's hope that this important door remains and stays open!

WHAT IS BUPRENORPHINE?

The purpose of chemistry is not to produce gold but to study the
basic sciences and use them against disease.

—Paracelsus

Figure 9

Suboxone Film

(Courtesy of Reckitt Benckiser)

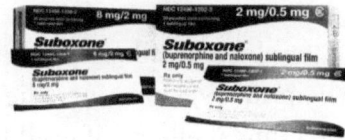

How should I take SUBOXONE sublingual film?

- Always take SUBOXONE exactly as your doctor tells you. Your doctor may change your dose after seeing how it affects you. Do not change your dose unless your doctor tells you to change it.
- Do not take SUBOXONE more often than prescribed by your doctor.
- Each SUBOXONE sublingual film comes in a sealed child-resistant foil pouch. Wait to open SUBOXONE until right before you use it.
- To open your SUBOXONE sublingual film foil pouch, fold along the dotted line and tear down at the slit (see Figure 1) or cut with scissors along the arrow.

Dosage Strengths

SUBOXONE Film is clinically interchangeable with SUBOXONE (buprenorphine and naloxone) sublingual tablets (CIII) and is available in 2 dosage strengths

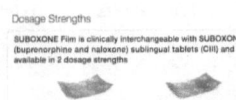

2 mg buprenorphine, 0.5 mg naloxone

8 mg buprenorphine, 2 mg naloxone

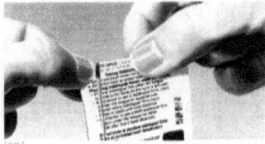

Figure 1

- Before taking SUBOXONE, drink water to moisten your mouth. This helps the film dissolve more easily.
- Hold the film between two fingers by the outside edges.
- **Place SUBOXONE sublingual film under your tongue,** close to the base either to the left or right of the center (see Figure 2).

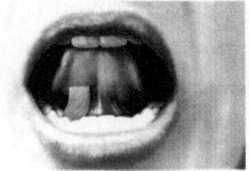

Buprenorphine is closer to the perfect substitution medication that we have in addictions.

Initially it was marketed as IM (intramuscular) analgesic (Bupronex) and approved by the FDA in 2002 as a sublingual tablet (now film) with buprenorphine only (Subutex). Or (Suboxone) with added Naloxone (which is an opiate blocker) to diminish risk of diversion. 2 mg of Suboxone has 0.5 of naloxone; 8 mg of buprenorphine has 2 mg of naloxone.

Now we think that with implanted buprenorphine, more persons addicted to opiates will get almost cured! In a recent interview, Dr. Volkov stated, "Implantable buprenorphine could improve outcomes for patients who abuse opioids or are addicted to heroin."

Their compliance and risk of diversion will certainly improve.

Suboxone is a sublingual film formulation for patients with opioid dependence. The primary active ingredient is buprenorphine. The other, naloxone, has no clinical effects; if used by mouth, it is almost nil. It has clinical effects of withdrawal if injected IV consequently discouraging diversion.

Bupronorphine has the following characteristics:

- It has high affinity for the μ-opioid receptor.
- Low intrinsic affinity, less euphoria, and ceiling dose to prevent respiratory depression.
- Slower dissociation means milder withdrawal profile.
- It is the first and only medication approved by the FDA for the office-based medical management of opioid addiction.
- It is long-acting, from 24-48 hours duration.
- Safe.
- Effective.

It will precipitate withdrawal if given too soon after ingestion of a pure opioid agonist.

Eight to twelve milligrams are usually sufficient to relieve withdrawal because about 86 percent of opioid brain receptors are filled with it. The longer the patient waits, the better it will work not less than twenty-four hours after the use of a full agonist like OxyContins. In the case of methadone, at least thirty-six hours after the last dose is taken, the subject should be on not more than 40 mg of methadone.

Pharmacokinetics

Bupronorphine is a partial µ-opioid agonist. The fact that it is a partial opioid agonist means it has a ceiling dose. In other words, it cannot cause respiratory depression and death by OD. Big difference and merit! After buprenorphine introduction in France, the number of deaths due to OD decreased by 70 percent.

It is approximately 96 percent bound in the plasma and undergoes N-dealkylation via the cytochrome P450 (CYP450) 3A4 enzyme system to produce and active metabolite norbuprenorphine. Both undergo glucoridation in the liver, and 30 percent of the drug is eliminated in urine and 70 percent in feces. Buprenorphine has a mean elimination half-life from plasma of thirty-seven hours. Its above metabolism means that other substances metabolized by the 3A4 system could raise levels (grape-fruit juice/fluoxamine, fluoxetine, sertraline, etc.), and inducers (carbamazepine/rifampin) could lower its levels. With the exception of some antiretroviral medications (nelfinavir), it looks like these interactions are of no clinical significance.

Deaths have been associated with injecting buprenorphine and benzodiacepines and other CNS depressants. Therefore, the use of sedative-hypnotics is a relative contraindication. For instance, Ambien and buprenorpohine. If needed, both doses should be lowered.

Side effects of buprenorphine can include constipation, nausea, and vomiting, but their frequency is much lower than with full opioid agonists. Patients maintained in buprenorphine show no clinically significant disruption in cognitive and psychomotor performance on formal testing.

Mild elevation after receiving sublingual buprenorphine levels of the liver enzymes alanine aminotransferase (ALT) and aspartate aminotransferase (AST) have been reported in patients treated for more than forty days. It was found that patients with a history of viral hepatitis were more likely to have these elevations in liver enzymes. It is important to note that these elevations were quite small and of questionable clinical significance. There are reports of very high transaminase elevations associated with intravenous buprenorphine in patients infected with the hepatitis C virus. The proposed mechanism is inhibition of hepatic mitochondrial function by very high buprenorphine concentrations associated with injection, but not with sublingual dosing. A recent communication about buprenorphine as part of Medical Support of Addiction Recovery by Scott A. Oakman, MD, (72) states that drugs affect the gene expression and connectivity to other neurons. The success he states of buprenorphine is due to the widespread of synthetic medical opioids (oxycodone). I disagree with his statement that buprenorphine "does not appear to reverse physical dependence." I think it does, and the good news is that in updated research, it has been proven to be superior to methadone among pregnant addicted persons. When appropriately used, it can be very successful.

The prescription of buprenorphine has two models:

- One is strict and follows methadone and the classic treatments of addiction with twelve-step meetings and close monitoring of the use of this medication as well as other addictive drugs. The attendance to twelve-step meetings is compulsory and should be documented and signed by the sponsor or other recovering person; counseling with a therapist or counselor is also mandatory. The induction or initial session takes care in the doctor's office for not less than 2-3 hours with UDS (urine drug screening), and weekly follow-ups at one, two, or four weeks (when the buprenorphine maintenance dose is established) is required and every visit thereafter. Finalized with the end-bupronorphine treatment as described below is indicated.

- The other model is more flexible—a real officelike model. Home-buprenorphine induction (73) in the first interview may be tried in the appropriate patient. Where flexibility does not mean permissiveness, which does not mean lack of patient's responsibility for their treatment. Patients have to attend the doctor's office at least monthly. UDS should be performed at random, and encourage as many supports as possible, but it shifts the responsibility to the patient.

According to some like Dr. George Kolodner (74), the UDS are more negative for other drugs or more positive for buprenorphine with the first model. However, I think that all depends on your sample. If the patient has strong motivation to stay clean and has a job, belongs to middle class, and has supports, the second model could be tried.

Clinical Use Issues

Four different clinical formulations of buprenorphine are available in the United States:

1. Suboxone (Reckitt Benkiser Labs), a buprhenorphine/naloxone combination in tablets and film of 2/0.5 mg/ 8/2mg respectively.
2. Subutex (Reckitt Benkiser Labs), just buprenorphine 2-8 mg for the use of pregnant women and detox only; it will be discontinued as of January 1, 2012.
3. Buprenex (generic buprenorphine by Ben Venue Laboratories, 2004), an injectable formulation of the schedule III narcotic (opioid); approved for the use as an analgesic; not approved for use in the treatment of opioid addiction. But it can be given for the

treatment of painful syndromes. 300 mcg/dose IM/IV q 6-8 h. Max 300 mcg/dose IV; 600 mcg/dose IM.

4. Butrans (buprenorphine transdermal by Perdue Labs), in 5, 10, 20 mcg/h patch approved only for pain, moderate to severe chronic. Max 20 mcg/h. 5-20 equivalent to 30-80 mg of morphine/daily.

Sublingual Forms

Sublingual buprenorphine is available in the United States in two forms. One is Suboxone, referred to as "the combo product" that combines buprenorphine and naloxone in a homogenous compressed film; the other is Subutex, referred to as "the mono product," a tablet that contains only buprenorphine. It is safe and effective. Children cannot open the film pouch. The film has a track number to discourage diversion. This formulation will be discontinued as of January 1, 2012.

The combo combination was designed to prevent diversion, first in a tablet form, now in film. There is research going on to develop a transdermal form. However, eye-contact with the doctor at least once a month plus all the ancillary support groups have a real salutary effect because they help establishing astral connections "the spiritual awakening" described above and should not be deleted or replaced for interventions less effective. The buprenorphine "diversion" keeps agents of the DEA occupied. With the threat of rescheduling buprenorphine into schedule II type of a drug, which means that then it will be used only in federally approved clinics similar to methadone maintenance. Nonetheless, the number of addicted person to opioids, more than two million, will be out of their reach! Nevertheless, I think that a more effective use of these DEA agents' time could be on the irresponsible and excessive use of Oxys and Xanax, which are rampant. The diversion of buprenorphine is mainly due to financial profit and the unprofessional treatment of withdrawal from opioids. Many take the buprenorphine too early, and it just precipitates a more intense withdrawal. The street value of buprenorphine could go as high as $ 20-40 per 8 mg film or tablet. Recently there was an isolated report in a New

Jersey jail of children coloring books tinted with buprenorphine? Needless to say not a successful business for drug dealers because it does not cause a real high and is not an effective way of administering it.

Office-Based Buprenorphine Treatment

(Available since November 2002 when Suboxone/Subutex were approved by the FDA and after the doctor takes appropriate training and obtains a DEA license)

The first step is to make the diagnosis of opioid addiction according DSM-IV or fulfilling the 3 C's of addiction as stated above. Then, the most important issue is to select the appropriate person to benefit from buprenorphine. (Remember buprenorphine is not for everybody.) These are guidelines. Nothing replaces the physician acumen to select the patient.

The optimal patient should have the following seven characteristics:

1. Strong motivation to quit opioids. The patient must understand that this medication will help him to prevent severe social-psychological consequences. It has a preventive feature. This medication is legal and approved by the FDA.
2. Not have polydrug addiction with especially strong addiction to benzodiacepines.
3. Low suicidal/homicidal risk profile.
4. Not in a methadone maintenance program.
5. Not pregnant. (In this case, methadone maintenance is the standard of treatment or Subutex.)
6. Not seek only buprenorphine as the main and only treatment of a painful syndrome.
7. Not have the diversion-like syndrome profile person: have a steady job or income with good and efficient supports that contributes to the enhancement of good outcome and astral connections.

Before selecting the patient. In-service staff training is essential. Buprenorphine treatment is a team effort. As such, all the staff should be on "the same page." The head of the team is the physician. The receptionist, UDS staff, therapists, counselors, up to the CEO, and others staff members must be part of this team. Consequently, all of them should participate or be aware of the in-service buprenorphine training. The limit setting that most patients need starts with their signature of a contract, which should be frequently reminded, and the reminder of ongoing REMS, plus UDS at random.

Adopting a new treatment modality can be challenging, especially to staff members who are not familiar with addictions or have the Semmelweis reflex reaction (narrow-minded or not understand that this is a different type of treatment) and consider all addicted patients as "just manipulative." Nothing can be further from the truth. One size does not fit them all. All depends on your comfort zone. One recommendation is, as Jefferson said, "Trust but verify." Not all addicted persons are the same nor the addicted to opiates. Some of them may need it as maintenance therapy. In this sense, I very much agree with Dr. Joseph Pinciotti's (75) division of five different options to end patients on buprenorphine. Remember that some patients may have a combination of these five types. Dr. Pinciotti is a well-experienced buprenorphine physician and speaker for Reckett Benckiser pharmaceutical company.

Suboxone End of Treatment Options

1. Some people take Suboxone for the prescribed minimum of 6-12 months; then they taper their dose, have no symptoms, and stop entirely.
2. Other patients taper after 6-12 months but choose to stay on a low dose as a blocker to prevent relapsing.
3. Those patient who have physical pain for various conditions may slowly feel their pain increases as their Suboxone dose decreases.

Since their medicine does confer moderate pain relief, they choose to remain on Suboxone as a pain relief (not approved by the FDA but can be given as off label).

4. With higher dosages of street drugs, they are individuals who have created a permanent damage to their brain receptors. They will experience drug cravings for a long time, possibly forever, and they must remain on Suboxone at a lower dose to prevent relapsing.

5. Certain underlying medical, mental conditions, such as bipolar disorders, ADHD, a mixture of depression and anxiety, can trigger relapse. One way of explaining this is that their receptors are genetically abnormal or imbalanced, and they will forever crave drugs if their receptors are not filled with something. These people are at very high risk of relapse without treatment with Suboxone as maintenance dose.

Dr. Pinciotti tells patients that "this is an oversimplification, but conveys a working knowledge of this medication as a tool." His five group patients division is a good clinical way to see that not all the patients are alike!

The need to expand treatment services is urgent and the potential to improve the lives of addicted persons is enormous.

Any office providing buprenorphine treatment should do it in a well-coordinated medical, psychiatric, or social treatment. Models for the treatment of chronic medical ailments such us diabetes offer some guidance. A nurse, a counselor, a clinical social worker, the secretaries or another nonphysician provider assumes a role in monitoring patients under the direction of the physician. It is a team approach!

In any shared model, physicians need to ensure that the amount of physician supervision and contact is safe, appropriate, and consistent with clinical guidelines, which as the name says, are just "guidelines" (an indication or outline of policy or conduct).

In this office model, the communication and coordination with other treatment providers is also essential. Accordingly, patients should sign a contract and information release forms compliant with the Health Insurance Portability and Accountability Act of 1996 (HIPAA). For instance, psychiatrists may require that a patient have a primary care physician. Making connections with specialty addiction treatment providers such as those that work with detoxification centers and in the methadone maintenance programs are particularly important.

Since some patients may resist treatment providers' efforts to communicate with each other because of fear, stigma, embarrassment, etc., some techniques to facilitate communication should be developed. These should be informed consent, short contracts or treatment planning, which should be frequently reminded, agreements or letters clarifying the intent of improving communication and avoiding duplication of treatment.

Discussing the length of opioid treatment is important. Most patients want short-term treatment. However, the longer the treatment, the better the outcome, and for many patients, indefinite treatment may be needed. It is important to give patients enough time to meet their treatment goals and enjoy the benefits of the investment they have made by engaging in treatment.

These two treatments office models complement the use of buprenorphine under the biopsychosocial model.

There is no doubt that professional counseling improves the outcome. This involves the assessment for professional treatment, the twelve-step model, residential and intensive outpatient programs.

Also, motivation enhancement therapy/facilitating involvement in twelve-step groups/cognitive behavior therapy (CBT) and end with relapse-prevention counseling.

Management of Acute and Chronic Pain in Opioid-Addicted Patients (76)

Because chronic pain is common among patients with comorbidity before buprenorphine was approved, we wanted to do some research with Dr. Irajd Maany who is also certified as a pain specialist at Brooke Glen Behavioral Treatment Hospital. However, due to logistic issues, we were not able to do so. Since buprenorphine has been used to treat pain and now is approved for the treatment of opioid addiction as common sense says, it should help both. However, some guidelines are as follows.

Pain Assessment

Since self-reporting remains the golden standard for assessing pain. On a 0-10 point scale, 1-3 is considered mild pain, 4-7 moderate pain, and severe pain over 7.

To understand the impact of chronic pain on function, other measures such as brief pain inventory (Tan et al., 2004). In addition, physicians should obtain information and results from prior pain evaluations, which will help make an accurate diagnosis.

For the treatment of acute and chronic pain, it must be remembered that patients need to be reassured that if possible, their maintenance therapy with buprenorphine should be continued.

1. If there is sudden discontinuation of buprenorphine, for instance due to surgery, consult with the surgeon. About 24-48 hours before surgery, replace with a full opioid agonist, such as Percocet. Caution should be taken if it is abruptly discontinued. Increased sensitivity to the use of full agonists with respect to CNS and respiratory depression could occur. Naloxone, as an opiate blocker, should always be available.

2. Gradual discontinuation of buprenorphine. Divide the buprenorphine dose and administer every 6-8 hours, that is, until all its analgesic effects last due to the lack of analgesic ceiling effect. However, due to the presence of a respiratory depression ceiling effect, it is possible to safely administer additional doses of buprenorphine up to 72 mg for acute pain gradual buprenorphine titrating its dose, and treat with schedule full opioid agonist analgesics (e.g., sustained-release and immediate-release morphine.) With resolution of the acute pain, discontinue the opioid agonist analgesics and resume buprenorphine maintenance (some advice to repeat the buprenorphine induction). It is important the patient should be in mild opioid withdrawal before restarting buprenorphine therapy. About twenty-four hours after the full agonist is discontinued (forty-eight hours at least in the case of methadone).

Another word of caution. It is not recommended to use mixed agonist-antagonistic opioid analgesics such as pentazocine (Yalwin), nalbuphine (Nubain), and butorfanol (Stadol); they are likely to displace the buprenorphine from the μ receptor and precipitate withdrawal.

Opioid analgesic combinations such as acetaminophen and an opioid (e.g., Percocet, Vicodin) should be limited to situations not requiring large doses so as to avoid acetaminophen-induced hepatotoxicity.

I will finalize and summarize the most common and current medications for the treatment of addictions.

CONCLUSIONS

There are two types of medications.

1. Those that interfere with the reinforcing effects of a drug (Disulfiram for alcohol/Naltrexone for opiates)
2. Those that compensate for the adaptations that either predated or developed after long-term use (When physical withdrawal develops, substitution therapies: benzodiacepines for alcohol and other sedative drugs, methadone/buprenorphine for opiates. The trade names are in parentheses.)

Clinical Target Medication (*FDA Approved)

Alcoholism
Disulfiram (*Antabuse)
Naltrexone (*Revia)
Acamprosate (*Campral)

Cocaine under Investigation
Topiramate (Topomax)
Gabapentin (Neurontin)
Baclofen (Lioresal)
Modafinil (Provigil)
Disulfiram (Antabuse)
Cocaine vaccine

Opiate Dependence
Methadone (*Dolophine)
Naltrexone (*Revia)
Buprenorphine (*Suboxone/Subutex)

Smoking Cessation
Nicotine replacement patch
Bupropion (*Wellbutrin)
Varenecicline (*Chantix)

Under investigation
Rimonabant (Acomplia)

I will reiterate the main goals of this book. The biopsychological model is the par excellence model. It is crucial in the treatment and prevention of addictions. Some of this model's limitations are that it does not explain too much about the probably more important factors of astral or spiritual changes (in the brain) that take place in a person who is recovering.

Buprenorphine is the best substitution medication we have so far in the treatment of opioid addictions, and we need more medications like buprenorphine or better. Not all the patients are the same, and every treatment plan should reflect this. The patients are the most important part of the disease, and they should assume more active responsibility in their treatment and prevention of persons at risk to get it.

We have to know and learn more about the astral or spiritual forces in addictions. We need to know more scientific ways to separate different patient who may respond to different types of treatment. (In a few more years, pharmacogenetics may be cost effective and useful.)

Finally, if our attitude toward persons who have this disease is done as an art and science, always treating them with respect, we will have achieved something so important that has not been achieved in two thousand years! However, it is better late than never.

Let me close with a tribute and recognition to the real champions of the addiction contest: the patients who succeed achieving and maintaining sobriety. They stop their destruction and put their above-average intelligence and efforts to good work. With the help of the biopsychosocial model, which implies the use of medication that replace their lack of endogenous neurotransmitters, positive social changes happen, and they become productive in their communities throughout psychological and *astral* or *spiritual* changes. It reminds me of what goes on with exercise (now much popular with the mushroom growth of many gyms and body-building facilities). For instance, in the athlete's mind, what separates great professional athletes from the good ones? (77) A profound mind-body-social connection that is achieved through rigorous physical, mental, and social training. Sometimes seven hours of biking and swimming daily! Good example of real perseverance! Do you want something more compulsive than that? Once the addicted persons succeed with their commitment to maintain their sobriety, they are just better at managing it. In this sense, there are real champions of humanity embracing the biopsychosocial model totally and applying it to stay sober. They have to persevere in this endeavor to the very end.

South Africa Archbishop Desmond Tutu's Message of Forgiveness

The highlight of the American Psychiatric Association meeting in Honolulu in May 2011 was Archbishop-emeritus Desmond Tutu's presentation that was spellbinding, provoking a thunderous applause. He said, "We are all family—there are no outsiders." When we embrace our humanity, racial and religious differences dissipate. Can we imagine a world where forgiveness is the rule? Nothing will be more welcome in these days of war. Thank God the war in Iraq is ending! Archbishop Tutu concluded, saying, "All are welcome: black, white, red, yellow, rich, poor, educated, not educated, male, female, gay, straight, all, all, all. We all belong to this family, this human family."

The contradiction of the drug addict as a bad person who has been punished and criminalized but deep down is a good person who needs to be treated with respect and admiration is portrayed in the movie *Biutiful* (2010) (orthographic Spanish spelling of "beautiful") where Javier Bardem, Oscar winner in the picture *No Country for Old Men* gives us the landscape of addiction and the tragedy of illegals (Chinese and Senegalese) in the underworld of Barcelona. The actor's contradiction living in the dangerous underworld (Bardem plays the person named Uxbal who has a bipolar wife also addicted to alcohol, two children wanting to go to a beautiful ("biutiful") place in the Spanish Pyrenees. It is a circular tale—it ends where it begins, connecting in the afterworld with his deceased father after Uxbald dies from terminal prostate cancer. Uxbal has also the power to communicate with the afterlife (thus with his father whom he never knew because when his mother was pregnant, his father escaped the Spain dictated by Franco's regime to Mexico, where he died, and his embalmed body was brought back to Barcelona).

Struggling between morality, love, and spirituality, illuminating the inheritance bestowed from father to child, his paternal hand navigating the corridors of bad or beautiful, he like our patients who are successful in staying sober with his spirituality (astral forces) reaches freedom and eternity, which is symbolized by the Celtic cross.

SAMHSA (Substance Abuse Mental Health Services Administration) has released a new definition of recovery. *Los Angeles Times* (12/30, Roan) and clarified four major dimensions: health, home, purpose, and community that support a life in recovery. "A process of change through which individuals improve their health and wellness, live a self-directed life, and strive to reach their full potential."

This definition could not have a better example than the following.

I will finish with a very happy note. I was invited to Arlene's silver anniversary of being clean for twenty-five years without one relapse! She had been addicted a quarter of a century ago. I was fortunate to have been called to help her, and I did. Of course, with the help of many other supports, especially her husband, she is a successful and productive editor in our society, who remains active in the recovery community. She is the inspiration to many. It was a real honor for me to have been invited to her twenty-fifth year celebration of being sober, on September 16, 2011. She inspires many others to follow her footsteps. That is the name of the game! No doubt in my mind that she has found the way through spirituality and the supernatural to keep her clean. Her invitation words were "on September 16, 2011, I will celebrate 25 years clean! It is quite a milestone. And though it is tempting to take total credit for this accomplishment, I know I had a lot of help along the way. You were there at the very beginning, and I can never thank you enough for your kindness, support, and guidance. Not only during my inpatient stay at Huntington Hospital, but also during those first crucial months back in society." She continues, "But more than anything I just want to thank you for being there to help me celebrate my anniversary. You can't possibly know how much that meant to me. It made the day even more special."

SUMMARY

This book starts with the Celtic cross as a symbol of faith and peace. It emphasizes the biopsychosocial medical model for the treatment and prevention of this chronic illness we call addiction versus criminalizing them. What we do not know enough is the spiritual or astral aspects of it, for instance, the use of acupuncture among addicted persons who may have several medical and psychiatric comorbidities. Hopefully in the future, we will.

Meantime, nothing replaces the physician acumen to select the appropriate patient for the appropriate type of treatment. "One size does not fit them all." Each addicted person is a challenge and different from the next one. To treat them with the utmost respect and acknowledging their suffering of a severe medical illness should be our motto.

It describes historical, genetic, and neurochemical as well as clinical aspects of the three more common addictions: alcohol, cocaine, and opiates. It also makes reference to their usefulness among nonaddicted persons where moderation is the name of the game.

It claims that buprenorphine is the best medication currently available for the treatment of opioid addiction, which should be used only in the appropriate patient plus all the supports available to help addicted persons achieve "a spiritual awakening," which will help them succeed in their recovery, becoming productive members in our society.

NOTES

1. http:/www.celtarts.com/celic.htm. 8/8/2011.
2. *Merriam-Webster's Dictionary and Thesaurus*. 2006 by Merriam-Webster, Incorporated.
3. Addictions Means Enslavement. Clean and Sober Daily News, Spring 1989.
4. Fabiani, C. The Disease of Addictions. MEDICO INTERAMERICANO. Year 7. No. 9, pp. 23-66. September 1988.
5. Weiss, P. Principles of Development. New York: Holt, 1939.
6. Bertalanffy, L. von. "General Systems Theory and Psychiatry" in pp. 705-721. New York: Basic Books, 1966.
7. Engel, G. L. The Need for a New Medical Model: A Challenge to Biomedicine. Science 1977; 196: 129-136.
8. Diagnostic and Statistical Manual of Mental Disorders, Fourth Edition. DSM-IV-TM pp. 181. American Psychiatric Association, 1400 K Street, NW, Washington, DC 2005.
9. The Definition of Addiction(Long Version). ASAM. www.asam.org?DefinitionofAddiction-Long Version.html. 8/16/2011.
10. http://www.paralumun.com/astral.htm. 8/3/2010
11. Fabiani, C. C., Spiritual Chats (Unpublished manuscript, 1977).
12. Dr. Bob and the Good Old Times, pp. 9-23. Alcoholic Anonymous Services, Inc. 1980.
13. "Fifty Years with Gratitude," Alcoholic Anonymous, World Services Inc., September 1985.
14. Cohen, S., Cocaine Anonymous. Drug Abuse and Alcoholism. NEWSLETTER Vol. XIII, No. 3. April 1984.

15. Fabiani, C. A., Delgado M., Multiple Diagnoses among Puerto Rican Latino Patients at APM, AAOP Journal: Spring 1992. Vol. 4, No. 2.

16. Fabiani, C. A., Arce, A. A., Trastornos Psyquiatricos coexistentes en Hispanos. MEDICO Interamericano. Enero 1997. Vol. 16 No.1.

17. Brenda Borell. What's so Hot About Chile Peppers? Smithsonian.com, March 19, 2009.

18. Gallup: 50 % Believe Marijuana Should Be Legal. APA Office of Communications and Public Affairs. 10/19/2011.

19. California Secretary of State. California Proposition 215: Text of proposed law. Available at: http://vote96.sos.ca.gov/Vote96/html/BP/ 215text.htm (accessed July 27, 2011). APA Office of Communications and Public Affairs. 11/01/10.

20. Coffee Associated with Lower Rates of Depression in Women. APA Office of Communications and Public Affairs. September 27, 2011.

21. "Injustice" REELZ TV Channel. 2008. Philadelphia 10/20/11.

22. *The Triumph of Bacchus* in *Art and Images in Psychiatry*. Section Editor: James C. Harris, MD. Arch Gen Psychiatry/VOL 68 (NO, 1) January 2011.

23. Psychiatric News, September 17, 2010.

24. Rush B., Inquiry into the Effects of Ardent Spirits upon the Human Body and Mind. College of Physicians. Philadelphia, 1785.

25. Trotter Thomas, An Essay, Medical, Philosophical, and Chemical, on Drunkenness and Its Effects on the Human Body. Printed for T. N. Longman, and Ress, Paternoster Row, London, 1804.

26. Jellinek, E. M., The Disease Concept of Alcoholism. Highland Park, New Jersey, Hillhouse Press, 1960.

27. Huss, M., Alcoholismus chronicus. Chroniskm alcoholisjudkom: Ett bidrag till dyskrasarnias kanndom. Stockholm: Bopnner/Norstedt, 1849.

28. Manual on Alcoholism of the American Medical Association, 1968.

29. Yamamoto et al. Alcoholism in Peru. Am Journal of Psychiatry 150: 1959-1060, 1993.

30. Kuszynski-Godard, M., Paz Soldan, C. E., Diseccion del indigenismo Peruano. Lima. Publicaciones del Instituto de Medicina Social. Univ. Mayor San Marcos, 1948.

31. Fabiani, C. A., Foulks, E. F., Bolivian Alcoholic Pseudotetany. Abstracts. VI World Congress of Psychiatry. Page 142. Honolulu, Hawaii 8/28-29/1977.

32. Fabiani, C. A. Tetania Alcoholica Boliviana. MEDICO Interamericano. pp. 9-18. Marzo 1986.

33. Fabiani, C. A., Actitudes y Adicciones.Medicina y Cultura. pp.11-12. Volumen XII/No. 3 Agosto de 2003.

34. Schuckit, M. A., Update on Alcoholism Audio-Digest Psychiatry. Vol. 39, Issue 08. April 21, 2010.

35. Franks, N. P., Lieb, W. R. Seeing the light: protein theories of general anesthesia. Anesthesiology 2004; 101: 235-237.

36. Snell, L. D., Nunley, K. R., Lickteig, R. L., et al. Regional and subunit specific changes in NMDA receptor mRNA and immunoreactivity in mouse brain following chronic alcohol ingestion. Mol Brain Res 1996; 40: 71-78.

37. Olds, J., Milner, P., Positive Reinforcement Produced by Electrical Stimulation of Septal Area and Other Regions of Rat Brain. J. Comp Physiol Psychol 1954: 47: 419-427.

38. Kendler, K. S. et al. A twin-family study of alcoholism in women. Am J Psychiatry 15(5): 707-715, 1994.

39. Ross et al. Age, Ethnicity, and Comorbidity in a National Sample of Hospitalized Alcohol-dependent Women Veterans. Psychiatric Services 49 (5), 1998.

40. Biomarker May Help determine Severity of Alcohol Dependence, pp. 15 Psychiatric News/November 18, 2011.

41. Jellinek, E., The Disease Concept of Alcoholism, 1966.

42. Babor, T. F., Caetano, R., Subtypes of substance dependence and abuse: implications for diagnostic classification and empirical research. Addiction 2006; 101 (suppl 1) : 104-110.

43. Willinbring, M. I., "Treatment of Heavy Drinking and Alcohol Use Disorders" In *Principles of Addiction Medicine, Fourth Edition*, pp 335-347. Wolters Kluver? Lippincott Williams & Wilkins, 2009.

44. Lloyd, G., One hundred alcoholic doctors: a 21-year follow-up. Alcohol Alcohol. 2002; 37(4): 370-374.

45. Niemann, A., Uber eine neue organische Base in den Coca blattern, Gottingen, 1860.

46. Diaz, Villamil A., "La Leyenda de la Coca," in *Las mejores leyendas y tradiciones de Bolivia*, Antonio Paredes.

47. Bandelier, A. F., Aboriginal trephining in Bolivia. Antropol 6 (4):July-September 1904.

48. Riveros, Tejada A., The Coca Nostra.Doc. La Paz, Bolivia 11/15/10.

49. Carter, W., Mamani, M. "Irpa Chico": Individuo y Comunidad en la cultura Aymara. La Paz, 1982.

50. Carter, W., Mamani, Pocoata. Uso Tradicional de la coca en Bolivia. America Indigena XXXVIII (4): 905-937, 1978.

51. Freud, S. "Uber Coca." Secundaratz. Im K. K. Allgemeinen. Krankehause in Wien. Centralblatt fur die ges. Therapie. 2, 289314, Juli 1884.

52. Byck, R. Cocaine Papers Sigmund Freud. New American Library, 1974.

53. Koller, Carl, "Personal Reminiscences of the First Use of Cocaine as a Local Anesthetic in Eye Surgery." Read at the Sixth Annual Congress of the Anesthetists of the United States and Canada in joint meeting with the International Anesthesia Research Society, VII, No. 1 January-February 1928.

54. Mantegazza, "Sulle virtu igieniche e medicinali della coca. Memoria onorata dell' Acqua nel concorso di 1885, estratto degli Annali Universali di Medicina 1959."

55. Stewart, F. E., Coca Leaf Cigars and Cigarettes. Medical Times. September 19, 1885.

56. TV6. ABC News 11 PM, Philadelphia. December 1, 2001.

57. Volkow, N. D., Li, Ting-Kai. "Drug Addiction: The Neurobiology of Behavior Gone Awry." Principles of Addiction Medicine pp. 3-12. 2009 by Lippincott Williams and Wilkins, a Wolters Kluwer business.

58. Leshner, A., "Addiction Is a Brain Disease, and It Matters." Sober Re-Sources: In Search of the Neurobiology of Addiction Recovery. September 6, 2007.

59. Volkov, N. D., Transforming Clinical Outcomes in Addiction Lecture #16. May 16. The 164th Annual Meeting of the American Psychiatric Association. Honolulu, Hawaii. 2011.

60. Noya, N. D., Coca and Cocaine Perspective from Bolivia. The International Challenge of Drug Abuse. NIDA Research Monograph 19, 1978.

61. Jeri, R., Del Pozo, T., Fernandez, M. El Sindrome De La Pasta de Coca. Revista De La Sanidad. De Las Fuerzas Armadas Policiales, 39, 1-18. 1978.

62. Opioid Overdose Quadrupled over Last Decade. December 2011. www.clinicalpsychiatrynews.com.

63. Benezet, A., A lover of mankind. Mighty Destroyer Displayed in some account of the dreadful havoc made by the mistaken use as well as abuse of distilled spirituous liquors. Philadelphia: Joseph Crukshank, 1974.

64. Renner, J. A., Levounis, P., Handbook of Office-Based Buprenorphine Treatment of Opioid Dependence. Opioid dependence in America. pp.1-21. American Psychiatric Publishing, Inc., 2011.

65. Physicians Key to Strategy for Reducing Opioid Abuse. Psychiatric News/ May 20, 2011.

66. Fishman, Scott M. Responsible Opioid Prescription. CME Activity Copyright 2009. The University of Wisconsin Board of Regents.

67. Dole, V. P., Nyswander, M. E., A Medical Treatment for Diacetyl-Morphine (Heroin) Addiction. JAMA 1965; 193-646.

68. Hser, Y. I., Hoffman, V., Grella, C. E., et al., A 33-year follow-up of narcotic addicts. Arch Gen Psychiatry 58: 503-508, 2001.

69. Psychiatric Pharmacogenomics, Psychiatric Times, December 2011. Vol. XXVIII. No. 12

70. Clinical Guidelines for the Use of Buprenorphine in the Treatment of Opioid Addiction. TIP 40. US Department of Health and Human Services. 2004.

71. Johnson, R. E., Buprenorphine Treatment. Holiday Hotel, Philadelphia, Pennsylvania 7/6/11.

72. Oakman, Scott A. Medical Support of Addiction Recovery. Audio-Digest Psychiatry. Volume 40, Issue 18. September 21, 2011.

73. Lee, J. D., Grossman, E., DiRocco, D., et al., Home buprenorphine/naloxone induction in primary care. J G Intern Medicine 24: 226-232, 2009.

74. Kolodner, G., Practical Suggestions for Improving Your Results Using Buprenorphine. pcssb@psych.org. September 13, 2011.

75. Pinciotti, jodeoh60@aol.com. Suboxone end of treatment. December 13, 2011.

76. Psychiatrists' Expertise Useful in Managing Chronic Pain. Psychiatric News/ pp. 18, June, 2011.

77. Inside an Athlete's Mind. DRIVE. pp. 12-16. The Magazine from Subaru. Summer 2011.

INDEX

I

J

K

L

M

N

O

V

W

www.ingramcontent.com/pod-product-compliance
Lightning Source LLC
Chambersburg PA
CBHW031302280526
45784CB00004B/1960